Workbook for
Nursing Assisting
A Foundation in Caregiving

THIRD EDITION

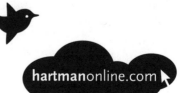

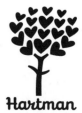

Credits

Managing Editor
Susan Alvare Hedman

Cover Designer
Kirsten Browne

Cover Illustrator
Jo Tronc

Production
Thad Castillo
Tak Minagawa

Proofreaders
Kristin Calderon
Kristin Cartwright

Copyright Information

© 2012 by Hartman Publishing, Inc.
8529 Indian School Road, NE
Albuquerque, New Mexico 87112
(505) 291-1274
web: hartmanonline.com
e-mail: orders@hartmanonline.com

ISBN 978-1-60425-031-2

PRINTED IN THE USA

Notice to Readers

Though the guidelines and procedures contained in this text are based on consultations with healthcare professionals, they should not be considered absolute recommendations. The instructor and readers should follow employer, local, state, and federal guidelines concerning healthcare practices. These guidelines change, and it is the reader's responsibility to be aware of these changes and of the policies and procedures of her or his healthcare facility.

The publisher, author, editors, and reviewers cannot accept any responsibility for errors or omissions or for any consequences from application of the information in this book and make no warranty, expressed or implied, with respect to the contents of the book. The publisher does not warrant or guarantee any of the products described herein or perform any analysis in connection with any of the product information contained herein.

Table of Contents

1. The Nursing Assistant in Long-Term Care   1

2. Ethical and Legal Issues   9

3. Communication Skills   17

4. Communication Challenges   27

5. Diversity and Human Needs and Development   33

6. Infection Prevention   39

7. Safety and Body Mechanics   45

8. Emergency Care, First Aid, and Disasters   51

9. Admission, Transfer, Discharge, and Physical Exams   55

10. Bedmaking and Unit Care   59

11. Positioning, Moving, and Lifting   63

12. Personal Care   67

13. Vital Signs   73

14. Nutrition and Fluid Balance   79

15. The Gastrointestinal System   89

16. The Urinary System   95

17. The Reproductive System   99

18. The Integumentary System   101

19. The Circulatory or Cardiovascular System   105

20. The Respiratory System   107

21. The Musculoskeletal System   111

22. The Nervous System   115

23. The Endocrine System   127

24. The Immune and Lymphatic Systems and Cancer   131

25. Rehabilitation and Restorative Care   135

26. Subacute Care   139

27. End-of-Life Care   143

28. Your New Position   149

Procedure Checklists   155

Practice Exam   229

Preface

This workbook is designed to help you review what you have learned from reading your textbook. For this reason, the workbook is organized around learning objectives, just like your textbook and even your instructor's teaching material. Including the learning objectives makes it easier for you to go back and reread a section if you need to refresh your memory.

These learning objectives work as a built-in study guide. After completing the exercises for each learning objective in the workbook, ask yourself if you can DO what that learning objective describes.

If you can, move on to the next learning objective. If you cannot, just go back to the textbook, reread that learning objective, and try again.

We have provided procedure checklists, as well as a practice exam for the certification test, at the end of the workbook. The answers to the workbook exercises are in your instructor's teaching guide.

Happy Learning!

1

The Nursing Assistant in Long-Term Care

1. Review the key terms in Learning Objective 1 before completing the workbook exercises

2. Describe healthcare settings

Multiple Choice
Circle the letter of the answer that best completes the statement or answers the question.

1. Another name for a long-term care (LTC) facility is:
   (A) Nursing home
   (B) Home health care
   (C) Assisted living facility
   (D) Adult daycare facility

2. People who live in long-term care facilities are called residents because:
   (A) The facility is their home.
   (B) They are picked up at the end of each day to go home.
   (C) They do not have any living family members.
   (D) They do not need skilled care.

3. Assisted living facilities are initially for:
   (A) Residents who need around-the-clock intensive care
   (B) Residents who are generally independent and do not need skilled care
   (C) Residents who will die within six months
   (D) Residents who need to be in an acute care facility

4. How does home health aide care differ from nursing assistant care?
   (A) Home health aides do not have to assist with personal care.
   (B) Home health aides may clean the home and do laundry.
   (C) Home health aides do not have supervisors.
   (D) Home health care takes place in a hospital, rather than in a long-term care facility.

5. A program of care given by a specialist or a team of specialists to restore or improve function after an illness or injury is called:
   (A) Acute care
   (B) Subacute care
   (C) Rehabilitation
   (D) Hospice care

6. Inter-generational care is:
   (A) People of the same generation spending time together
   (B) Pets brought into the facility to help brighten a resident's day
   (C) Adult and child daycare merged so that young and old can spend time together
   (D) The generation caring for children and aging parents at the same time

3. Explain Medicare and Medicaid

True or False
Mark each statement with either a "T" for true or an "F" for false.

1. _____ Medicare is a health insurance program for people who are 65 years of age or older.

2. ____ No one younger than 65 is covered by Medicare.

3. ____ Medicare will pay for any services requested by the resident.

4. ____ A person with limited income might qualify for Medicaid.

5. ____ Medicare and Medicaid pay a fixed amount for services based on residents' needs.

4. Describe the residents for whom you will care

True or False

1. ____ It is more important to know residents individually than to know general facts about most residents.

2. ____ Most residents living in long-term care facilities are male.

3. ____ Residents with the longest average stay in a healthcare facility are residents admitted for rehabilitation or terminal care.

4. ____ Dementia is not a major cause of admission to a long-term care facility.

5. ____ Poor health is not the only reason residents are admitted to long-term care facilities. Often they are admitted due to lack of a support system.

6. ____ Lack of outside support is one reason to care for the "whole person" instead of only the illness or disease.

5. Describe the nursing assistant's role

Short Answer
Answer each of the following questions in the space provided.

1. What are activities of daily living (ADLs)?

_____

_____

_____

_____

2. Think of one task that might be assigned to a nursing assistant that is not mentioned in the book.

_____

_____

_____

_____

_____

3. List seven tasks performed by nursing assistants. Which task do you think you will enjoy the most? Which do you think will be the hardest for you?

_____

_____

_____

_____

_____

_____

_____

_____

_____

_____

_____

6. Discuss professionalism and list examples of professional behavior

Multiple Choice

1. Which of the following shows professionalism?
   (A) It is okay to arrive late or leave early; if a nursing assistant is not there during scheduled times, her coworkers can cover for her.
   (B) A nursing assistant should never discuss personal problems with residents.
   (C) The way a nursing assistant dresses is unimportant.
   (D) Accepting tips from residents is a good idea because it makes up part of a nursing assistant's salary.

2. Katie is a new nursing assistant at Parkwood Skilled Nursing Care and wants to make a good first impression. What is one thing she can do to show professionalism at her new job?
   (A) Ignore any constructive criticism she receives from others.
   (B) Tell a resident about another resident's condition in order to gain the resident's trust.
   (C) Ask questions when she does not understand something.
   (D) Address the residents by using affectionate nicknames like "Honey" or "Granny."

7. List qualities that nursing assistants must have

Scenarios
Read each of the following scenarios and answer the questions that follow.

Nursing assistant Samantha Stevens is late for five shifts in a row. On the fifth day, her supervisor asks her about this. Samantha replies, "It's not my fault. Traffic has been horrible, and I just wish this facility was on a more convenient street."

1. How could Samantha have been more humble and open to growth?

   _____

   _____

   _____

   _____

   _____

   _____

   _____

Nurse Frederico Gonzalez tells nursing assistant Mary Lupko about a resident's diagnosis of a sexually-transmitted disease. He gives specific instructions about the resident's care. Mary sees a fellow nursing assistant across the hall, and says, "How do you think Joann Timbly got an STD? Her husband hasn't visited in months."

2. How could Mary have been more trustworthy?

   _____

   _____

   _____

   _____

   _____

   _____

   _____

Nursing assistant Rob Brown is tidying Ms. Lee's room. He notices a Buddha statue and asks, "Why don't you believe in Christ? Christianity is the only real religion."

3. How could Rob have acted in a courteous and respectful manner?

   _____

   _____

   _____

   _____

   _____

Resident Hannah Stein is dying. She tells nursing assistant Jennifer Wells that she always wanted to be nicer to her son and to have a better relationship. Jennifer replies, "Yeah, well, you think you got it hard? My son won't even talk to me because I wouldn't let him go to a basketball game on a school night." Then Jennifer proceeds to tell Mrs. Stein about her divorce and how her son's father never helps out.

4. How could Jennifer have been more empathetic?

   _____

   _____

   _____

   _____

   _____

_____
_____
_____
_____
_____

Nursing assistant Doug Albin is helping resident Sam Perkins to the bathroom. Sam walks slowly and has to rely on his walker for help. Doug notices that his shift is over in five minutes. Doug says, "Can't you walk a little faster? I'm outta here in five minutes!"

5. How could Doug have been more patient and understanding?

_____
_____
_____
_____
_____
_____
_____

Nursing assistant Wayne Leach just found out his facility is short-staffed tonight, and he will have to help five additional residents get ready for bed. "Oh great," he says. "Now I'll never get this done!"

6. How could Wayne have been more enthusiastic?

_____
_____
_____
_____
_____
_____
_____

Nurse Cathy Connell verbally gives nursing assistant Sandra Levy a list of things she wants done. Sandra simply says, "Okay" and walks off. As she turns the corner, she forgets what Nurse Connell wanted her to do first. "Oh well," she shrugs. "I'm sure it's not the end of the world."

7. How could Sandra have been more dependable?

_____
_____
_____
_____
_____
_____
_____
_____
_____
_____
_____

Nursing assistant Tracy Fleming is assigned to help Mr. Ming, a resident from China, eat his dinner. Even though she has never met Mr. Ming, she complains, "I can never understand anything these kinds of residents are saying."

8. How could Tracy have been more tolerant and unprejudiced?

_____
_____
_____
_____
_____
_____
_____

8. Discuss proper grooming guidelines

True or False

1. _____ Long hair should be kept down around the face while giving care to residents.

2. _____ False nails harbor bacteria no matter how well hands are washed.

3. _____ Wearing strong scents or perfumes at work is a good idea.

4. _____ Hoop earrings can be worn around residents who will not pull them out.

5. _____ A nursing assistant should wear light makeup or none at all.

6. _____ Long nails are fine to have, as long as they're not false nails.

7. _____ Jewelry can collect bacteria.

8. _____ A nursing assistant only needs to bathe or shower three times a week.

9. Define the role of each member of the care team

Matching
Write the letter of the correct description beside each care team member listed below. Use each letter only once.

1. _____ Registered dietician

2. _____ Physician

3. _____ Occupational therapist

4. _____ Medical social worker

5. _____ Activities director

6. _____ Speech-language pathologist

7. _____ Nurse

8. _____ Resident

9. _____ Nursing assistant

10. _____ Physical therapist

(A) Person who determines residents' needs and helps them get support services, such as counseling and financial assistance

(B) Person who is the most important part of the care team

(C) Person who gives therapy in the form of heat, cold, massage, ultrasound, electricity, and exercise to improve circulation, promote healing, ease pain, and improve mobility

(D) Person who performs many assigned tasks, such as bathing residents, and assisting with toileting; the person who usually has the most direct contact with residents

(E) Person who teaches exercises to help residents improve or overcome speech problems; also evaluates ability to swallow food and drink

(F) Person who assesses residents, creates the care plan, monitors progress, and gives treatments

(G) Person who diagnoses disease or disability and prescribes treatment

(H) Person who assesses the resident's nutritional status and plans a program of nutritional care

(I) Person who works with people who need help with activities of daily living

(J) Person who plans activities for residents to help them socialize and stay active

10. Discuss the facility chain of command

Fill in the Blank
Fill in the correct word in each blank below.

1. The chain of command describes the line of _____ in a facility.

2. The _____ will usually be the nursing assistant's immediate supervisor.

3. When a nursing assistant has a problem with another department, it should be reported to an immediate supervisor or the _____ nurse.

4. Following the chain of command protects staff from _____, which is a legal term for being held responsible for harming someone else.

_____

_____

_____

11. Explain "The Five Rights of Delegation"

Short Answer

1. What are three questions nurses consider before delegating a task?

_____

_____

_____

_____

_____

_____

_____

_____

_____

_____

_____

_____

2. What are three questions nursing assistants should ask themselves before accepting a delegation?

_____

_____

_____

_____

_____

_____

_____

_____

3. If a nursing assistant is unsure about a task that is delegated to him, what should he do?

_____

_____

12. Describe four methods of nursing care

Matching
Use each letter only once.

1. ____ Team nursing

2. ____ Functional nursing

3. ____ Resident-focused care

4. ____ Primary nursing

(A) Method of care which is based upon a partnership between the residents, their families, and their caregivers

(B) Method of care in which a nurse acts as the team leader of a group of individuals giving care

(C) Method of care assigning specific tasks to each team member

(D) Method of care in which the registered nurse gives much of the daily care to residents

13. Explain policy and procedure manuals

Fill in the Blank

1. A _____ is a course of action to be taken every time a certain situation occurs.

2. A complete list of every facility policy is found in the _____.

3. A _____ is a specific way of doing something.

4. The exact way to complete every resident procedure is found in the _____.

5. Nursing assistants who _____ when they are unsure provide safer care.

14. Describe the long-term care survey process

True or False

1. _____ A survey is conducted by a team of professionals to make sure long-term care facilities are following state and federal regulations.

2. _____ If a surveyor asks a nursing assistant a question and the nursing assistant does not know the answer, she should quickly make one up to avoid being cited.

3. _____ Surveyors will interview residents to get their opinions about the care they receive.

4. _____ Membership in the Joint Commission is mandatory for all healthcare facilities.

2

Ethical and Legal Issues

1. Review the key terms in Learning Objective 1 before completing the workbook exercises

2. Define the terms "law," "ethics," and "etiquette"

Multiple Choice

1. The knowledge of right and wrong are:
   (A) Ethics
   (B) Civil laws
   (C) Etiquette
   (D) Criminal laws

2. Which of the following is a law?
   (A) A nursing assistant must not gossip about residents or other staff members.
   (B) A nursing assistant must be polite when answering the telephone.
   (C) A nursing assistant must not steal residents' belongings.
   (D) A nursing assistant must not discuss personal problems with co-workers.

3. Laws to protect individuals from people or organizations that try to do them harm are:
   (A) Civil laws
   (B) Criminal laws
   (C) Felonies
   (D) Misdemeanors

4. A code of courtesy and proper behavior in a certain setting is called:
   (A) Civil law
   (B) Criminal law
   (C) Ethics
   (D) Etiquette

3. Discuss examples of ethical and professional behavior

Crossword Puzzle

Across

1. Treating residents with this means allowing others to believe or act as they wish to do

2. Being able to share in and understand the feelings of others

5. Another word for private (resident information must remain _____)

6. Nursing assistants must refuse these when they are offered

Down

1. If a nursing assistant makes a mistake, it is important to do this immediately

3. Being this way means that a nursing assistant is able to speak and act without offending others

4. Ways that a nursing assistant can demonstrate being _____ include being truthful when reporting hours and documenting care accurately

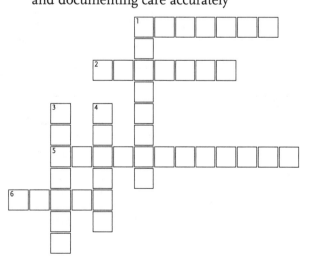

4. Describe a nursing assistant code of ethics

Short Answer

1. What is one way that a nursing assistant can make sure she keeps up with new information on the job?

_____

_____

_____

_____

_____

2. What are two ways you plan to show a positive attitude toward residents, staff, and visitors when you start your new job?

_____

_____

_____

_____

_____

_____

_____

_____

3. What is one way to help preserve resident safety?

_____

_____

_____

_____

_____

_____

4. If a nursing assistant suspects that a resident is being abused, what should she do?

_____

_____

_____

_____

_____

5. Explain the Omnibus Budget Reconciliation Act (OBRA)

Multiple Choice

1. Why was the Omnibus Budget Reconciliation Act (OBRA) passed in 1987?
   (A) As a response to reports of poor care and abuse in long-term care facilities
   (B) Because of complaints of uncooperative residents by nursing assistants
   (C) To control costs in long-term care facilities
   (D) Because most long-term care facilities employed too many nursing assistants

2. How does the OBRA law relate to nursing assistants?
   (A) Tests nursing assistants' knowledge of care procedures
   (B) Sets minimum requirements for training, competency exams, and in-service education
   (C) Outlines specific steps for handling infectious material
   (D) The OBRA law does not apply to nursing assistants

3. How many hours of training must nursing assistants complete before working to meet OBRA requirements?
   (A) 30 hours
   (B) 50 hours
   (C) 75 hours
   (D) 100 hours

4. Which of the following is a part of OBRA's regulations?
   (A) OBRA establishes the correct steps to follow if a nursing assistant is exposed to a bloodborne pathogen.
   (B) OBRA requires assessments only for residents with certain medical conditions.
   (C) OBRA details the safe use of and hazards of chemicals.
   (D) OBRA requires standardized training of nursing assistants.

6. Explain Residents' Rights

Short Answer

For each of the following Residents' Rights, give one example of how a nursing assistant can respect that right while working.

1. The right to the best quality of life possible

_____

_____

_____

_____

_____

_____

2. The right to receive the correct care in the form of services and activities to maintain a high level of wellness

_____

_____

_____

_____

3. The right to be fully informed about rights and services

_____

_____

_____

_____

_____

4. The right to participate in their own care

_____

_____

_____

_____

_____

5. The right to make independent choices

_____

_____

_____

_____

_____

6. The right to privacy and confidentiality

_____

_____

_____

_____

7. The right to dignity, respect, and freedom

_____

_____

_____

_____

_____

8. The right to security of possessions

_____

_____

_____

_____

_____

9. Rights with transfers and discharges

_____

_____

_____

_____

_____

10. The right to complain

_____

_____

_____

_____

_____

11. The right to visits

_____

_____

_____

_____

_____

_____

12. Rights with regard to social services

_____

_____

_____

_____

_____

_____

7. Explain types of abuse and neglect

Matching
Use each letter only once.

1. ____ Abuse
2. ____ Active neglect
3. ____ Assault
4. ____ Battery
5. ____ Domestic violence
6. ____ False imprisonment
7. ____ Financial abuse
8. ____ Involuntary seclusion
9. ____ Negligence
10. ____ Passive neglect
11. ____ Physical abuse
12. ____ Psychological abuse
13. ____ Sexual abuse
14. ____ Sexual harassment
15. ____ Substance abuse
16. ____ Verbal abuse
17. ____ Workplace violence

(A) Actions, or a failure to act or give proper care, that results in injury to a person

(B) The use of legal or illegal drugs, cigarettes, or alcohol in a way that is harmful to the abuser or to others

(C) Any unwelcome sexual advance or behavior that creates an intimidating or hostile work environment

(D) Intentionally harming a person physically, mentally, or emotionally by failing to give needed or correct care

(E) Separating or confining a person from others against the person's will

(F) The unlawful restraint of someone which affects the person's freedom of movement

(G) Verbal, physical, or sexual abuse of staff by residents, other staff members, or visitors

(H) Touching a person without his or her permission

(I) The act of threatening to touch a person without his or her consent

(J) The act of stealing, taking advantage of, or improperly using the money, property, or other assets of another

(K) Forcing a person to perform or participate in sexual acts

(L) The use of language—spoken or written—that threatens, embarrasses, or insults a person

(M) Any behavior that causes a person to feel threatened, fearful, intimidated, or humiliated in any way

(N) Physical, sexual, or emotional abuse by spouses, intimate partners, or family members

(O) Causing physical, mental, emotional, or financial pain or injury to someone

(P) Intentional or unintentional treatment that causes harm to a person's body

(Q) Unintentionally harming a person physically, mentally, or emotionally by failing to give needed or correct care

Multiple Choice

1. What should a nursing assistant do if he sees or suspects that a resident is being abused?
   (A) Report it to the supervisor and document it at once.
   (B) Keep watching the resident to make sure he is correct.
   (C) Ignore it until the resident complains about it.
   (D) Confront the abuser.

2. If a resident wants to make a complaint of abuse, the nursing assistant's responsibility is to:
   (A) Confirm that abuse has really occurred before reporting it.
   (B) Assist the resident in every possible way.
   (C) Retaliate against the resident for making a complaint.
   (D) Ask other residents if they have seen any abuse occurring.

3. An example of sexual abuse is:
   (A) A nursing assistant does not respond to a call light.
   (B) A nursing assistant shows a resident a pornographic magazine.
   (C) A nursing assistant leaves a resident alone in his room and does not check on him.
   (D) A nursing assistant screams at a resident.

4. An example of financial abuse is:
   (A) A nursing assistant loudly announces in the hallway that a resident has "wet his bed again."
   (B) A nursing assistant makes fun of a resident's religion.
   (C) A nursing assistant sells crafts that a resident has made for profit and keeps the money.
   (D) A nursing assistant hits a resident.

5. An example of psychological abuse is:
   (A) A nursing assistant roughly hurries a resident to the bathroom.
   (B) A nursing assistant tells a resident he needs money for school.
   (C) A nursing assistant forces a resident to rub up against her.
   (D) While giving care to a resident, a nursing assistant tells him he smells bad.

8. Recognize signs and symptoms of abuse and neglect

True or False

1. _____ Ignoring a call light is not considered abuse or neglect.

2. _____ Unexplained broken bones, burns, and bruising are all signs of abuse.

3. _____ Lack of appetite and weight loss can be signs of abuse.

4. _____ Similar injuries that occur over and over probably just mean that the resident is clumsy.

5. _____ If a resident shows fear or anxiety when a certain caregiver is present, this may be a sign of abuse.

6. ____ Mood swings and depression are always caused by illness or chemical imbalance.

7. ____ If a resident is unclean or has a strong smell of urine, it probably just means he does not like to bathe.

8. ____ Sores on the body can indicate neglect.

9. ____ If a resident's family is concerned that abuse is occurring, it is considered a possible sign of abuse.

10. ____ If a nursing assistant only suspects abuse, she should wait until she is sure it is happening before reporting it.

9. Describe the steps taken if a nursing assistant is suspected of abuse

Multiple Choice

1. What is the first thing that happens when a report of nursing assistant abuse has been made?
   (A) The NA is immediately fired.
   (B) The NA is immediately suspended.
   (C) The NA is allowed to keep working until the investigation is completed.
   (D) The NA is transferred to another facility.

2. Which of the following is a step taken by the Nurse Aide Training and Competency Evaluation Program (NATCEP) after a claim of abuse against a nursing assistant has been made?
   (A) An investigation is performed.
   (B) The nursing assistant is put in jail.
   (C) The resident is relocated to another facility.
   (D) All mail delivered to the facility is opened and searched.

3. If the claim of abuse is proven to be true, what happens?
   (A) The NA is placed in the abuse registry in addition to other possible penalties.
   (B) The resident is moved to another facility.
   (C) The NA is transferred to another facility.
   (D) The facility is cited for negligence.

10. Discuss the ombudsman's role

Short Answer

1. What is the role of an ombudsman?

_____
_____
_____
_____
_____
_____
_____
_____
_____
_____
_____

2. Which other people or organizations can a resident or his family contact for help or to make a complaint?

_____
_____
_____
_____
_____
_____

11. Explain HIPAA and related terms

Multiple Choice

1. Why was the Health Insurance Portability and Accountability Act (HIPAA) created?
   (A) To protect the privacy of health information
   (B) To reduce instances of abuse in facilities
   (C) To address infection prevention issues
   (D) To ensure adequate training for nursing assistants

2. Who may have access to private health information (PHI) about a resident?
   (A) Anyone who asks
   (B) Only the resident's friends and family
   (C) Only people who must have the information for care or to process records
   (D) No one

3. If a person who is not directly involved in a resident's care asks a nursing assistant for PHI, how should the nursing assistant respond?
   (A) Ignore them.
   (B) Ask the supervisor what to tell them.
   (C) Say, "I cannot share that information. It is confidential."
   (D) Tell them, but ask them not to tell anyone about it.

4. Which of the following is a way to keep private health information confidential?
   (A) Discussing residents' care outside of the facility, in public areas
   (B) Posting information to your Facebook wall
   (C) Only discussing residents with your family or friends
   (D) Properly disposing of notes regarding residents before you leave work

5. Which of the following is considered an invasion of a resident's privacy?
   (A) A nursing assistant tells her supervisor that she thinks a resident is starting to develop a pressure ulcer.
   (B) A nursing assistant shows her husband a photo of a new resident in her care.
   (C) A nursing assistant documents a resident's complaint of pain.
   (D) A nursing assistant refuses to share information about a famous resident with her neighbor.

6. A law that was enacted as a part of the American Recovery and Reinvestment Act of 2009 and helps expand the protection and security of consumers' electronic health records (EHR) is called:
   (A) HISEAL
   (B) HITECH
   (C) HIHELP
   (D) HIQUIET

12. Discuss the Patient Self-Determination Act (PSDA) and advance directives

True or False

1. _____ A DNR order tells healthcare professionals to keep trying to resuscitate a resident if his heart stops.

2. _____ The Patient Self-Determination Act encourages people to make decisions about advance directives.

3. _____ Advance directives designate the kind of care people want in the event they are unable to make those decisions themselves.

4. _____ A living will designates the people who will inherit the resident's estate if he or she dies.

5. _____ A durable power of attorney for health care appoints a person to make medical decisions for a resident if he or she becomes unable to do so.

6. _____ Facilities are required by Medicare and Medicaid to give residents and staff information about rights relating to advance directives.

3

Communication Skills

1. Review the key terms in Learning Objective 1 before completing the workbook exercises

2. Explain types of communication

True or False

1. _____ People communicate with words, drawings, pictures, and behavior.

2. _____ The receiver and sender never switch roles during communication.

3. _____ Speaking and writing are two examples of verbal communication.

4. _____ How a person's voice sounds and the words he chooses are not important during communication.

5. _____ Nonverbal communication includes posture and facial expressions.

6. _____ Making positive changes in body language will improve communication.

7. _____ It is a good idea for a nursing assistant to finish a resident's sentences for him to show that she understands what he is telling her.

8. _____ Use mostly facts when communicating with the care team.

Short Answer
For each of the following behaviors, decide whether it's an example of positive or negative nonverbal communication. Write "P" for positive or "N" for negative.

1. _____ Smiling

2. _____ Crossing arms in front of you

3. _____ Looking away while someone is talking

4. _____ Leaning forward to listen

5. _____ Pointing at someone while speaking

6. _____ Rolling eyes

7. _____ With permission, putting a hand over a resident's hand while listening to her

8. _____ Tapping a foot

9. _____ Nodding while a person is speaking

3. Explain barriers to communication

Scenarios
Read the scenarios below and answer the questions.

Nursing assistant Barbara Smith thinks resident Mrs. Gold is in pain. Barbara asks her if she is okay. Before Mrs. Gold answers, Barbara looks around the room and begins to gather her supplies to leave. Mrs. Gold simply says, "Yes."

1. Identify the barrier to communication occurring here and suggest a way to avoid it.

_____

_____

_____

_____

_____

_____

_____

_____

_____

_____

Resident Marla Gibson had a stroke that affects her speech. She asks her nursing assistant for a glass of water. The nursing assistant replies, "I'm not sure where your daughter is," and leaves the room.

2. Identify the barrier to communication occurring here and suggest a way to avoid it.

_____

_____

_____

_____

_____

_____

_____

_____

_____

_____

Nursing assistant Kena Wright asks resident Josiah Crane, "You have NKA, right?" He nods. She reports to the nurse, who looks over his chart. "No, that's not true," the nurse says. "He is allergic to penicillin. I wonder why he told you that."

3. Identify the barrier to communication occurring here and suggest a way to avoid it.

_____

_____

_____

_____

_____

_____

_____

_____

_____

_____

Nursing assistant Jerry Wells sees that resident Eli Levine is having difficulty moving his leg after his total hip replacement surgery. Jerry says, "You should start doing range of motion exercises right away and begin bearing as much weight as possible." Mr. Levine attempts to stand on his leg and screams in pain.

4. Identify the barrier to communication occurring here and suggest a way to avoid it.

_____

_____

_____

_____

_____

_____

_____

_____

_____

_____

Resident Paul Jackson is at risk for dehydration. Nursing assistants are asked to encourage him to drink as much as possible. To find out what Mr. Jackson likes to drink, nursing assistant Gracie Truman asks him, "Do you like orange juice?" He says, "No."

5. Identify the barrier to communication occurring here and suggest a way to avoid it.

_____

_____

_____

_____

_____

_____

_____

_____

_____

_____

Nursing assistant Lyla Cooper is helping resident Josie Bayer get ready to attend a guest lecture with another resident. Josie says, "I don't want to go with her." Lyla asks, "Why not?" Josie replies, "I just don't."

6. Identify the barrier to communication occurring here and suggest a way to avoid it.

_____

_____

_____

_____

_____

_____

_____

_____

_____

Nursing assistant Tracy Fleming is assigned to give Mr. Perez, who speaks very little English, a bed bath. She explains the procedure, and Mr. Perez nods even though he looks a little confused. When she starts to take off his shirt, he gets very upset.

7. Identify the barrier to communication occurring here and suggest a way to avoid it.

_____

_____

_____

_____

_____

_____

_____

_____

_____

4. List ways that cultures impact communication

Multiple Choice

1. Which of the following is true of cultures?

    (A) There are only a few cultures in the world.

    (B) The use of touch is the same for all cultures.

    (C) A culture is a set of learned beliefs, values, and behaviors.

    (D) The use of eye contact is the same for all cultures.

2. If a resident seems to be sensitive to eye contact and/or touch, a nursing assistant should:

    (A) Make eye contact and touch him as much as possible so that he gets used to it.

    (B) Respect his wishes and limit eye contact and touch as much as possible.

    (C) Explain to the resident that we do things differently in our culture, and he needs to adapt.

    (D) Ignore the sensitivity and use eye contact and touch as with any other resident.

3. Which of the following is a type of unacceptable touch when working with residents?

    (A) Sitting on a resident's lap

    (B) Cleaning a resident's arm during a bed bath

    (C) Hugging with permission

    (D) Holding a resident's hand if asked

4. One good way for a nursing assistant to deal with a language barrier with a resident is to:

    (A) Use an interpreter

    (B) Teach the resident words in the nursing assistant's language

    (C) Speak with other staff in the nursing assistant's language in front of the resident

    (D) Get someone else to care for the resident

Name: _____

5. Identify the people you will communicate with in a facility

True or False

1. ____ When a nursing assistant first greets a resident, he should introduce himself and identify the resident.

2. ____ In the facility, a nursing assistant may communicate by charting, using a computer, or on the telephone.

3. ____ If a nursing assistant has performed a procedure for a resident before, she doesn't need to explain it the next time she does it.

4. ____ Communication with other departments within a facility is not common and is unimportant.

5. ____ One way to let a resident's family know that staff are providing excellent care for him or her is to always answer call lights promptly.

6. ____ Families can provide valuable information about a resident's preferences and histories.

7. ____ If a doctor's office calls and asks for information about a resident, the nursing assistant should give it to them.

6. Understand basic medical terminology and abbreviations

Matching
Use each letter only once.

1. ____ Abbreviation

2. ____ Root

3. ____ Suffix

4. ____ Prefix

(A) The main part of a word

(B) A word part placed at the end of a word

(C) A word part added to the beginning of a word

(D) A shortened word

Short Answer

1. When is it appropriate to use medical terminology on the job? When is it inappropriate?

_____

_____

_____

_____

_____

_____

_____

_____

_____

2. How will knowledge of the abbreviations used in a facility make a nursing assistant's job easier?

_____

_____

_____

_____

_____

_____

_____

_____

_____

_____

7. Explain how to convert regular time to military time

Fill in the Blank
Fill in the correct time in each of the blanks.

Regular Time	Military Time
_____ p.m.	1500

5:00 p.m.   _____

_____ a.m.   0600

8:30 p.m.   _____

_____ p.m   1925

2:15 a.m.   _____

8. Describe a standard resident chart

Multiple Choice

1. When charting, the nursing assistant's role is limited to which of the the following?
    (A) Making changes in residents' diets
    (B) Changing medications
    (C) Gathering information and reporting to the nurse
    (D) Creating a new exercise plan

2. Which of the following is true of a resident's medical chart?
    (A) Care plans are not usually included in the medical chart.
    (B) Nursing assistants write their diagnoses in the medical chart.
    (C) Information about the resident's room-mate is included in the medical chart.
    (D) Doctors' and nurses' notes are included in the medical chart.

9. Explain guidelines for documentation

True or False

1. ____ A medical chart is a legal document.

2. ____ Information in a resident's chart may be shared with anyone who asks for it.

3. ____ It is appropriate to chart care before it has been performed.

4. ____ A nursing assistant should write his initials in pencil after each note he makes in the chart.

5. ____ When documenting, use only facts.

6. ____ If an error is made while document-ing, cross it out by drawing big circles through it.

7. ____ Use accepted abbreviations and terms when documenting.

10. Describe the use of computers in documentation

Word Search
Fill in each of the blanks and find your answers in the word search.

1. Computers can easily store information that can be _____ when needed.

2. Using a computer for charting is faster and more _____ than writing by hand.

3. Some facilities have a computer in every res-ident's _____.

4. Do not share your personal
    _____ or
    _____ ID
    with anyone.

5. Do not access _____ e-mail accounts or inappropriate _____ from work.

6. _____ privacy guidelines apply to computer use.

```
e  k  g  a  v  s  a  d  a  i  c  g  b  c
g  s  j  s  f  t  y  e  a  e  f  s  n  q
g  l  u  n  q  i  m  v  v  b  l  g  f  y
v  g  e  l  k  o  h  e  m  p  q  b  o  k
w  p  l  n  m  e  r  i  e  c  x  p  a  r
r  z  i  w  h  s  d  r  o  w  s  s  a  p
m  q  m  a  g  g  s  t  x  b  m  e  p  w
j  h  n  m  t  o  n  e  w  q  b  t  i  g
s  g  y  l  n  z  z  r  t  j  n  y  h  b
q  l  a  a  k  a  l  o  g  i  n  h  q  f
z  m  l  i  c  c  x  o  w  z  s  y  z  e
w  i  a  u  y  k  a  m  d  h  u  b  w  u
y  e  a  s  f  k  m  f  h  s  a  i  e  b
j  o  n  d  f  y  q  g  y  x  v  l  v  w
c  e  e  s  u  z  e  m  k  w  b  t  l  o
k  h  n  l  q  c  w  i  j  i  z  c  g  z
f  n  d  h  p  r  a  v  g  x  i  m  f  n
l  q  y  i  k  v  g  e  u  v  f  l  m  f
a  g  n  c  o  m  l  r  i  z  c  j  s  s
k  c  u  y  l  c  y  j  r  e  s  f  z  z
```

Name: _____

11. Explain the Minimum Data Set (MDS)

Multiple Choice

1. The Minimum Data Set (MDS) was created to:
   (A) Give facilities a structured, standardized approach to care
   (B) Give facilities more flexibility in how care is performed
   (C) Improve infection prevention in facilities
   (D) Help train nursing assistants

2. For which of the following situations does an MDS need to be completed?
   (A) When a resident leaves the facility
   (B) Once every five years after the first MDS has been completed
   (C) When there have been no major changes in a resident's condition for two weeks
   (D) Within 14 days of a resident's admission

3. What is the nursing assistant's role regarding the MDS?
   (A) Completing the MDS for each resident
   (B) Reminding the nurse when the MDS needs to be done
   (C) Reporting on changes in residents' health that may trigger a needed assessment
   (D) Deciding how to address problems discovered in the assessment

12. Describe how to observe and report accurately

True or False

1. _____ Any change in a resident's condition that is not serious does not need to be reported.

2. _____ Nursing assistants may notice more changes in residents than other care team members because they spend the most time with residents.

3. _____ Changes in a resident's condition that endanger residents should be reported right away.

4. _____ Nursing assistants make decisions regarding residents' health.

5. _____ Critical thinking for nursing assistants means the ability to make careful observations.

6. _____ A care plan is a written plan for each resident that outlines the steps and tasks needed to help the resident achieve his or her goals.

7. _____ Care plans are created by nursing assistants.

8. _____ Changes in a resident's weight do not need to be reported unless they are over 10 pounds.

Short Answer

For each of the following, decide whether it is subjective data (the resident must tell you about it) or objective data (data you collect using your senses). Write "O" for objective or "S" for subjective.

1. _____ Red streaks on skin

2. _____ Swollen foot

3. _____ Nausea

4. _____ Itchy arm

5. _____ Dizziness

6. _____ Fever

7. _____ Vomiting

8. _____ Chest pain

Short Answer

1. What is the nursing assistant's role in planning resident care?

_____

_____

_____

_____

_____

_____

_____

_____

_____

_____

2. For each of these four senses, list two observations that a nursing assistant might make using that sense.

• Sight

_____

_____

_____

_____

• Hearing

_____

_____

_____

_____

• Touch

_____

_____

_____

_____

• Smell

_____

_____

_____

_____

3. List three other ways to observe residents accurately.

_____

_____

_____

_____

_____

_____

_____

_____

4. List five signs and symptoms that should be reported immediately.

_____

_____

_____

_____

_____

_____

_____

_____

13. Explain the nursing process

Matching
Write the letter of the correct description beside each step of the nursing process. Use each letter only once.

1. _____ Assessment

2. _____ Diagnosis

3. _____ Planning

4. _____ Implementation

5. _____ Evaluation

(A) In agreement with the resident, goals are set, and a care plan is created to meet the resident's needs

(B) A careful examination to see if goals were met or progress was achieved

(C) Getting information from many sources to identify actual and potential problems

(D) Putting the care plan into action; giving care

(E) The identification of health problems after looking at all of the resident's needs

14. Discuss the nursing assistant's role in care planning and at care conferences

Multiple Choice

1. The purpose of a care conference is:
   (A) To train nursing assistants in new care skills
   (B) To decide how to remove a resident from a facility
   (C) To share and gather information about residents to develop a plan of care
   (D) To orient new residents to the facility

2. What is the nursing assistant's role at a care conference?
   (A) Keeping order at the meeting
   (B) Sharing observations gathered from resident care
   (C) Writing down the care plan
   (D) Explaining the care plan to the resident and family

3. If a nursing assistant is not sure what to say at a care conference, she should
   (A) Not attend the conference
   (B) Attend the conference but not say anything
   (C) Talk to the nurse before the conference to find out what she should say
   (D) Ask other team members at the meeting what information to share

15. Describe incident reporting and recording

True or False

1. ____ It is okay to change the facts a little when writing an incident report.

2. ____ Incident reports do not need to be completed if the injury is a small one.

3. ____ An incident is an accident, problem, or unexpected event that is not part of the normal routine of care.

4. ____ An incident report should be completed as soon as possible after the incident occurs so that details are not forgotten.

5. ____ The information in an incident report is available to the public.

6. ____ Both facts and opinions are included in an incident report.

16. Explain proper telephone etiquette

Multiple Choice

1. An example of proper telephone etiquette is:
   (A) Immediately putting the caller on hold without asking
   (B) Identifying the facility to the caller
   (C) Telling the caller, "Now is not a good time to call."
   (D) Giving the caller any information she asks for about residents and staff

2. Which of the following is a general rule for telephone use at a facility?
   (A) All facilities allow the use of cell phones at work.
   (B) Staff information can be disclosed to creditors if they call.
   (C) Resident information can be given to anyone who calls and inquires.
   (D) Resident information cannot be given over the phone.

17. Describe the resident call system

Short Answer

1. What is the purpose of the facility call system?

   _____

   _____

   _____

   _____

   _____

   _____

2. Why is answering a resident's call light promptly so important?

   _____

   _____

   _____

   _____

_____

_____

_____

(C) Tasks that are done for residents every day

(D) Advanced life support provided to a resident during an emergency

18. Describe the nursing assistant's role in change-of-shift reports and "rounds"

Fill in the Blank

1. Examples of information passed on to the next shift are _____ that occurred, appetite problems, difficulties with urination, complaints of _____, or a change in the ability to _____.

2. At start of shift reports, listen to important information about all of the _____ in the area.

3. Special information shared during a report may include new _____ and transfers or _____ from the facility.

4. Before the end of shift report, tell the nurses about such things as changes in _____ or temperature and skin changes that could signal the start of a _____ _____.

5. A method of reporting where staff members move from room to room and discuss each resident and the plan of care is called _____.

19. List the information found on an assignment sheet

Matching

1. _____ Code

2. _____ Code status

3. _____ Range of motion

4. _____ Activities of daily living

(A) Exercises done to bring joints through a full range of movement

(B) Tells whether a resident has an advance directive or not

20. Discuss how to organize your work and manage time

Crossword Puzzle
Across

4. Talking with residents while providing care is an example of _____ activities

5. Identify the most important things to get done and do those first

6. Being able to ask for this when needed is important

Down

1. These should be located within a resident's reach before a nursing assistant leaves him or her

2. Doing this with duties helps nursing assistants complete their assignments each day

3. Making one of these involves writing out the hours of the day and filling in when a nursing assistant will do what

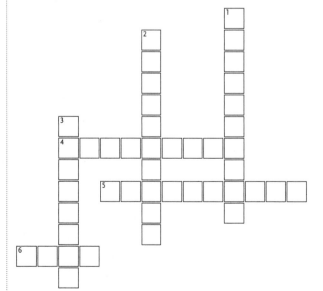

4

Communication Challenges

1. Review the key terms in Learning Objective 1 before completing the workbook exercises

2. Identify communication guidelines for visual impairment

Word Search

1. A(n) _____
    is a partial or complete loss of function or
    ability.

2. _____ and
    _____ are two diseases that
    can cause visual impairment.

3. Do not _____
    a person with a visual impairment before
    speaking to him or her.

4. Make sure there is proper
    _____ in the room.

5. Do not _____.

6. Use the face of an imaginary
    _____
    to explain the position of objects.

7. If the resident has _____
    make sure they are clean and fit properly.

8. Do not move personal items or
    _____
    without the resident's permission.

9. Read _____ to the resident.

10. Do not play with or distract
    _____.

11. Be _____
    and try to imagine what it feels like to not be
    able to see well.

```
e  i  y  m  t  v  j  m  o  a  e  g  u  o
v  c  b  u  e  i  w  b  j  d  r  l  k  w
u  q  o  w  t  n  s  j  j  m  u  a  x  z
k  h  b  i  d  f  u  i  r  s  t  u  v  l
s  q  z  v  c  i  g  s  z  c  i  c  d  q
t  n  e  m  r  i  a  p  m  i  n  o  h  b
e  d  z  i  w  w  t  b  s  u  r  m  c  e
v  k  l  j  c  o  s  e  e  i  u  a  u  t
x  f  f  y  g  v  r  e  h  t  f  v  o  u
g  u  i  d  e  d  o  g  s  t  e  q  t  b
g  n  i  t  h  g  i  l  j  s  a  s  l  i
l  c  y  x  y  j  y  r  l  m  a  p  d  z
c  l  o  c  k  h  e  s  l  j  n  l  m  c
f  n  w  w  w  c  b  y  v  r  a  c  g  e
```

3. Identify communication guidelines for hearing impairment

Multiple Choice

1. Which of the following is a symptom of
    hearing loss?
    (A) Trouble hearing high-pitched noises
    (B) Trouble hearing vowels
    (C) Being able to understand the meaning of
        words
    (D) Being able to hear people who are out-
        side of the room

2. Guidelines for communication with some-
    one who has a hearing impairment include:
    (A) Exaggerate pronunciation of words
    (B) Cover the mouth with a hand while
        speaking
    (C) Chew gum while speaking
    (D) Use simple words and short sentences

3. Which of the following is a way to help a person with a hearing impairment communicate more effectively?
   (A) Have a loud radio on in the room
   (B) Look away from the person while speaking
   (C) Be familiar with any hand gestures the person uses
   (D) Approach the person from behind

4. Explain defense mechanisms as methods of coping with stress

True or False

1. _____ Defense mechanisms allow a person to release tension or cope with stress.

2. _____ Repression means seeing feelings in others that are actually feelings within oneself.

3. _____ Displacement means transferring a strong feeling to a less threatening object.

4. _____ Defense mechanisms help a person to face the reasons a situation has occurred.

5. _____ Denial is rejecting a thought or feeling.

6. _____ Regression is making excuses to justify something.

5. List communication guidelines for anxiety or fear

Short Answer

1. Define anxiety.

_____

_____

_____

_____

2. List four physical symptoms of anxiety.

_____

_____

_____

_____

_____

_____

_____

3. List five guidelines for communicating with an anxious resident.

_____

_____

_____

_____

_____

_____

_____

6. Discuss communication guidelines for depression

True or False

1. _____ Losses that a resident may be experiencing include the loss of a spouse, friends, and independence.

2. _____ Depression can be managed, but it cannot be cured.

3. _____ One behavior that is associated with depression is a lack of interest in activities.

4. _____ Depression may be caused by a chemical imbalance.

5. _____ Most people who are depressed could choose to be well if they wanted to.

6. _____ It is never a good idea to touch a resident who is depressed.

7. _____ Do not talk to adults as if they were children.

8. _____ Depressed residents will never want to talk about their feelings.

9. _____ Signs of depression should be reported right away.

7. Identify communication guidelines for anger

Fill in the Blank

1. _____
   is a natural emotion that may be expressed by residents, their families and friends, and staff.

2. Loss of _____
   can cause a resident's anger.

3. Narrowed _____ and
   clenched or raised _____
   are signs of anger.

4. Anger may also be expressed by withdrawing or being _____.

5. If a resident's anger requires more time from staff, a _____
   may be scheduled.

6. When dealing with an angry resident, try to find out what _____
   the resident's anger.

7. Do not _____
   with the resident.

8. Try to involve the resident in
   _____.

9. _____ means
   being confident in dealing with other people. _____
   means expressing oneself in a way that humiliates or overpowers another person.

8. Identify communication guidelines for combative behavior

Multiple Choice

1. Which of the following should a nursing assistant do when dealing with combative behavior?
   (A) Call for the nurse immediately.
   (B) Get as close as she can to the resident.
   (C) Respond to insults with humor or sarcasm.
   (D) Threaten the resident if the behavior does not stop.

2. A nursing assistant's responsibility when a resident becomes combative is to:
   (A) Leave the resident alone.
   (B) Tell the resident that he is upsetting everyone and needs to stop.
   (C) Keep other people at a safe distance.
   (D) Restrain the resident if he does not calm down.

3. Under what circumstances may a nursing assistant hit a resident?
   (A) Any time a resident becomes combative
   (B) If the resident threatens to hit the nursing assistant
   (C) Only if the resident actually hits the nursing assistant
   (D) Never

9. Identify communication guidelines for inappropriate sexual behavior

Crossword Puzzle

Across

2. Nursing assistants must not do this regarding residents' sexual behavior

5. A nursing assistant should not

   _____

   when encountering an embarrassing situation, but instead should remain professional and calm.

6. The act of touching or rubbing sexual organs in order to give oneself or another person sexual pleasure

Down

1. Removing these in public areas is one example of inappropriate sexual behavior

3. One illness that can cause inappropriate sexual behavior

4. What a nursing assistant should provide if she witnesses consenting adults in a sexual situation

Name: _____

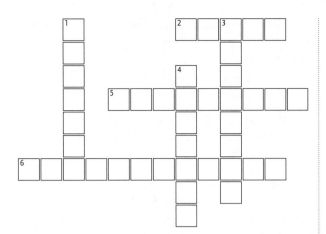

10. Identify communication guidelines for disorientation and confusion

Short Answer

1. Define disorientation and confusion.

_____
_____
_____
_____
_____
_____
_____
_____

2. List three things that a resident who is oriented should be able to tell the nursing assistant.

_____
_____
_____
_____
_____
_____
_____
_____

3. Name five physical problems that may cause confusion.

_____
_____
_____
_____
_____
_____
_____
_____

4. What are three things a nursing assistant can do to create a more comfortable environment for a resident who is confused?

_____
_____
_____
_____
_____
_____
_____
_____
_____
_____
_____

5. How can a nursing assistant make tasks easier for a person who is disoriented or confused?

_____
_____
_____
_____
_____
_____
_____

11. Identify communication guidelines for the comatose resident

Multiple Choice

1. Which of the following is true of a person who is in a coma?
   (A) A person in a coma is conscious.
   (B) A person in a coma can respond to changes in the environment, including pain.
   (C) A person in a coma may be able to hear what is going on in the room.
   (D) A nursing assistant should not speak to a person in a coma.

2. Which of the following should a nursing assistant try to do when caring for a resident who is in a coma?
   (A) Explain each procedure that the nursing assistant will be performing to the resident.
   (B) Hold personal conversations with others in the room since the resident cannot respond.
   (C) Remain silent at all times to avoid disturbing the resident.
   (D) Avoid touching the resident.

12. Identify communication guidelines for functional barriers

Fill in the Blank

1. Some things that can interfere with the ability to speak include difficulty in _____, physical problems with the _____ or _____, or an artificial _____.

2. If a resident has difficulty breathing, never push the resident to _____.

3. Birth defects such as cleft _____ may make speech difficult.

4. A(n) _____ is an opening through the neck into the trachea that is surgically created.

5. Ask the resident to _____ anything that is not understood.

6. Do not remove a resident's _____ for any reason.

7. Always report mouth sores and complaints of mouth pain, as well as poorly fitting _____.

8. Be _____ to the resident's situation by imagining how it might feel to have a tube in the nose, mouth or throat.

5

Diversity and Human Needs and Development

1. Review the key terms in Learning Objective 1 before completing the workbook exercises

2. Explain health and wellness

Short Answer

1. Define health and wellness.

_____

_____

_____

_____

_____

_____

_____

_____

_____

2. What is the focus of health?

_____

_____

_____

_____

_____

_____

_____

_____

3. For each of the five types of wellness, think of one thing that a nursing assistant can do to help residents achieve wellness in that area.

_____

_____

_____

_____

_____

_____

_____

_____

_____

_____

_____

_____

_____

_____

_____

_____

3. Explain the importance of holistic health care

Multiple Choice

1. Holistic care involves:
    (A) Dividing a system into parts
    (B) Caring only for a person's physical needs
    (C) Caring only for a person's psychosocial needs
    (D) Caring for the whole person

2. Which of the following is an example of a psychosocial need?
(A) Need for food
(B) Need to nurture spirituality
(C) Need to be free from pain
(D) Need for shelter

3. Which of the following is a good example of giving holistic care to a resident?
(A) Asking a resident to talk about her day while giving her a bath
(B) Rushing a resident through dinner to get tasks done more quickly
(C) Choosing a resident's clothes for him so he doesn't have to worry about it
(D) Trying to convert a resident to the nursing assistant's religion

4. Identify basic human needs and discuss Maslow's "Hierarchy of Needs"

Fill in the Blank

1. A _____ is something necessary for a person to survive and grow.

2. Residents need to feel as if they

_____ in their new home.

3. The first needs nursing assistants help residents meet are _____ needs like food and water, rest, and sleep.

4. Moving a person from her home into a facility can cause _____.

5. Residents may feel less of a sense of self-worth as they become

_____ on others.

6. The highest need a person can achieve, according to Maslow, is _____

_____.

5. Identify ways to accommodate cultural differences

True or False

1. ____ A nursing assistant will not need an understanding of different cultures to care for residents.

2. ____ Culture and background do not affect the way people behave when they are ill.

3. ____ A nursing assistant should respond to new ideas with acceptance rather than prejudice.

4. ____ People of all cultures tend to be embarrassed about discussing their health.

5. ____ Ask residents and their friends and families about their traditions and customs to give better care.

6. ____ If a resident does not understand the language the nursing assistant is speaking, the nursing assistant does not need to explain care procedures she is going to perform.

6. Discuss the role of the family in health care

Multiple Choice

1. Which of the following is true of families?
(A) There are "right" and "wrong" kinds of families.
(B) Families play an important role in residents' health care.
(C) Unmarried couples should not be considered a type of family.
(D) Families should not be allowed privacy for visits with residents.

2. When should staff become involved with family issues?
(A) Throughout the resident's stay in the facility
(B) Whenever the family has disagreements
(C) When there is concern about a resident's safety around family members
(D) Never

3. Which of the following is an example of a nuclear family?
(A) A mother, a father, and a child
(B) A mother, a father, a grandfather, and a child
(C) An uncle, a friend, and one parent
(D) A cousin, an aunt, and a child

4. When residents have visitors, a nursing assistant should:
   - (A) Do everything possible to help the resident prepare for the visit
   - (B) Ignore the visitors
   - (C) Tell the resident's family funny stories about him
   - (D) Watch the family closely to make sure the resident is not abused during the visit

7. Explain how to meet emotional needs of residents and their families

Crossword Puzzle

Across

3. Staff members who are prone to this are at risk for inappropriate relationships with residents

4. The care team member that families should be referred to when they ask nursing assistants about a resident's diagnosis

5. Nursing assistants must maintain these when working with residents and their families

6. Examples of one of these include "Everything will be fine" and "It all works out in the end."

Down

1. Nursing assistants can answer questions asked by residents and their families as long as the questions are within the NA's

   _____

2. It is important that nursing assistants listen and not do this when residents go to them with their problems

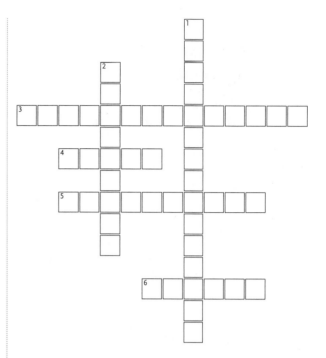

8. Explain ways to help residents with their spiritual needs

True or False

1. ____ A resident's religious items must be handled carefully.

2. ____ Respecting religious beliefs includes telling Muslim residents about Christianity.

3. ____ Spiritual needs are different for each person.

4. ____ Some people consider themselves spiritual but do not believe in a higher power.

5. ____ Residents who do not believe in God will not feel as strongly as residents who do.

Matching
Write the letter of the correct description beside each term related to religious faith or belief. Use each letter only once.

1. ____ Islam

2. ____ Buddhism

3. ____ Hinduism

4. ____ Judaism

5. ____ Atheism

6. ____ Christianity

7. ____ Agnosticism

(A) The Five Pillars of this religion include ritual prayer five times daily and donations to the poor and needy

(B) Baptism and communion may be part of this religion's practices

(C) Believe that they do not know or cannot know if God exists

(D) Believe that a person can reach Nirvana, the highest spiritual plane, after traveling through birth, life, and death

(E) Believe that actions in this life and past lives can determine one's destiny in future lives

(F) Believe that God gave them laws and commandments through Moses in the form of the Torah

(G) Actively deny the existence of God

9. Identify ways to accommodate sexual needs

True or False

1. ____ Most residents do not have sexual needs.

2. ____ Sexual identity does not play a very important role in a person's life.

3. ____ A transsexual person wishes to be accepted by society as a member of the opposite sex.

4. ____ Elderly people are not interested in sex.

5. ____ Illness may affect how a resident expresses himself sexually.

6. ____ Any expression of sexuality by older people is either disgusting or cute.

7. ____ If a nursing assistant encounters a resident engaging in a sexual activity, she should provide privacy.

8. ____ Residents have the right to choose how to express themselves sexually.

9. ____ If a nursing assistant sees a resident being sexually abused, she should not report it because it might embarrass the resident.

10. ____ Gay and lesbian are preferred terms when referring to people who are homosexual.

Short Answer

1. Gilda and Samantha both live in a care facility. Gilda is widowed, and Samantha has never been married. They met when Gilda was admitted six months ago. Gilda and Samantha have been sitting at the same table to eat their meals since Gilda moved in. Recently they have started spending time watching TV and playing cards in the day room together. Yesterday they took a walk outside. Linda, a nursing assistant, was gazing out the window and noticed them holding hands. Then she saw them stop behind the building and share a quick kiss. What are some responses that would respect Samantha's and Gilda's dignity and rights?

_____

_____

_____

_____

_____

_____

_____

2. Mr. Ramirez has a private room. His wife lives quite a distance away and only visits once every two weeks. The last time she visited, she requested a dinner tray and asked for both meals to be brought to his room. When Linda went to his room to deliver the meals, the door was shut. She walked in without knocking, and found them kissing each other in bed. She quickly exited the room and almost dropped the food on her way out. What could Linda have done differently? What should she do now that there has been an embarrassing moment?

_____

_____

_____

_____

_____

_____

_____

_____

3. List and describe six terms that define sexual identity.

_____

_____

_____

_____

_____

_____

_____

_____

_____

4. What are two reasons for a lack of sexual expression in long-term care facilities?

_____

_____

_____

_____

5. List four ways to help residents with their sexual needs.

_____

_____

_____

_____

_____

_____

_____

_____

_____

_____

_____

_____

_____

10. Describe the stages of human growth and development

Fill in the Blank

1. _____ refers to physical changes that can be measured.

2. _____ means the emotional, social, and physical changes that occur in a person's life.

3. _____ development is the process of gaining an ability to do such things as walking, drawing, and grasping.

4. _____ development is the process of children forming a sense of right and wrong.

5. _____ development focuses on how children think and learn.

6. _____ development is the process of learning to relate to other people.

7. _____ development has to do with the reproductive changes that occur when young people reach puberty.

Multiple Choice

1. In which stage of development is playing dress-up in parents' clothing common?
    (A) Toddler
    (B) Preschool
    (C) Adolescence
    (D) Infancy

2. Both genders become fully sexually mature during:
   (A) School-age
   (B) Adolescence
   (C) Middle adulthood
   (D) Late adulthood

3. Decisions about education, employment, and marriage often occur during this stage:
   (A) Young adulthood
   (B) Middle adulthood
   (C) Late adulthood
   (D) Adolescence

4. Which of the following is true of late adulthood?
   (A) People no longer need to stay connected to others.
   (B) People in this stage do not need to remain active.
   (C) People often retire from jobs and may need more medical care.
   (D) People undergo very few changes during this stage of life.

11. Discuss stereotypes of the elderly

Multiple Choice

1. Making a biased generalization based on false beliefs about a group is:
   (A) Stereotyping
   (B) Ageism
   (C) Opinions
   (D) Discrimination

2. Which of the following is a common stereotype about the elderly?
   (A) Elderly people have a sharp memory.
   (B) Elderly people are sexually active.
   (C) Elderly people are less intelligent than younger people.
   (D) Elderly people are very independent.

3. Most older people:
   (A) Do not like to leave home
   (B) Are active and have many interests
   (C) Cannot manage their money
   (D) Are ill and dependent

12. Discuss developmental disabilities

True or False

1. ____ Developmental disabilities are present at birth or emerge during childhood.

2. ____ Developmental disabilities can be cured.

3. ____ Developmental disabilities cause difficulty with language, learning, and self-care.

4. ____ The most common developmental disability is autism.

5. ____ People with developmental disabilities prefer to be treated like children.

6

Infection Prevention

1. Review the key terms in Learning Objective 1 before completing the workbook exercises

2. Define "infection prevention" and discuss types of infections

Matching
Use each letter only once.

1. ____ Communicable disease

2. ____ Cross-infection

3. ____ Healthcare-associated infection (HAI)

4. ____ Infection prevention

5. ____ Localized infection

6. ____ Microorganism

7. ____ Pathogen

8. ____ Reinfection

9. ____ Resistance

10. ____ Systemic infection

(A) A tiny living thing not visible without a microscope

(B) Infection that moves throughout the body

(C) The body's ability to prevent infection and disease

(D) Microorganism that is capable of causing infection and disease

(E) Infection that is limited to a specific part of the body

(F) The physical movement or transfer of harmful bacteria from one person, object, or place to another, or from one part of the body to another

(G) An infectious disease transmissible by direct contact or by indirect contact

(H) Being infected again with the same pathogen

(I) Set of methods used to control and prevent the spread of disease

(J) Infection associated with healthcare delivery in any setting, such as long-term care facilities and ambulatory settings

3. Discuss terms related to infection prevention

True or False

1. ____ Sterilization means all microorganisms are destroyed, including those that form spores.

2. ____ Medical asepsis means that a facility is completely free from all microorganisms.

3. ____ You must wash your hands before entering a clean utility room.

4. ____ Transmission is the process of removing pathogens.

5. ____ An object can be called "clean" if it has not been contaminated with pathogens.

6. ____ Spore-forming organisms, a special group of organisms that produce a protective covering that is difficult to penetrate, are killed by disinfection.

7. _____ Clean and dirty equipment, linen, and supplies are stored in the same utility room.

4. Describe the chain of infection

Short Answer

1. What does the chain of infection describe?

   _____

   _____

   _____

   _____

   _____

   _____

2. How many links in the chain of infection must be broken for infection to be prevented?

   _____

3. List the links of the chain of infection.

   _____

   _____

   _____

   _____

   _____

   _____

5. Explain why the elderly are at a higher risk for infection

Multiple Choice

1. One reason that older people are at a greater risk for acquiring infections is:
   (A) Their immune systems are stronger.
   (B) They are hospitalized more often.
   (C) Elderly people recover more quickly from illness.
   (D) Infections are less dangerous in older people.

2. Which of the following is a factor associated with aging that increases the risk of infection?
   (A) Thicker skin
   (B) Increased circulation
   (C) Use of catheters and other tubing
   (D) Increased mobility

6. Describe Centers for Disease Control and Prevention (CDC) and explain Standard Precautions

Fill in the Blank

1. The abbreviation for the government agency that promotes public health and safety and attempts to control and prevent disease:

   _____.

2. The two levels of precautions in the infection prevention system recommended by the CDC are Standard Precautions and

   _____

   _____.

3. Standard Precautions means treating all blood, body fluids, non-intact skin, and mucous membranes as if they were

   _____.

4. You cannot tell by looking at residents or their charts if they have a(n)

   _____ disease.

5. Wear a _____
   and protective _____ if
   you may come into contact with splashing or spraying body fluids.

6. Razor blades and other sharps should be disposed of in a _____
   container.

7. Never transfer _____
   items or any kind of _____
   from one room to another.

8. Never place _____
   items on the overbed table.

9. When cleaning anything, move from the
   _____ to the
   _____ area.

7. Define "hand hygiene" and identify when to wash hands

True or False

1. ____ Handwashing is the single most important method to reduce the spread of infection.

2. ____ Bacteria can be removed from artificial nails with thorough handwashing.

3. ____ Use of unscented lotions reduces risk of broken skin on hands.

4. ____ A nursing assistant must wash her hands every time she removes her gloves.

5. ____ A nursing assistant must wash his hands after he blows his nose.

6. ____ A nursing assistant does not need to wash her hands before obtaining clean linen from a cart.

7. ____ Use friction for no more than five seconds while washing hands.

8. ____ Using alcohol-based hand rubs means that nursing assistants do not need to wash their hands with soap and water.

8. Discuss the use of personal protective equipment (PPE) in facilities

True or False

1. ____ PPE is not important in preventing transmission of disease.

2. ____ The type of PPE a nursing assistant wears depends on what kind of exposure may be encountered.

3. ____ Gowns have to be worn if you may come into contact with splashing or spraying blood or body fluids.

4. ____ Gowns do not need to be changed if they become soiled or wet.

5. ____ Masks can prevent microorganisms from being inhaled.

6. ____ Masks should fit snugly over the nose and mouth.

7. ____ Special PPE will be required for a resident with tuberculosis.

8. ____ Disposable gloves can be washed and reused once they are clean.

9. ____ Gloves can be worn outside of a resident's room when a nursing assistant needs to grab something quickly.

Short Answer
Make a check mark (✓) next to the tasks that require you to wear gloves.

1. ____ Contact with body fluids

2. ____ Hanging laundry

3. ____ When you may touch blood

4. ____ Brushing a resident's hair

5. ____ Assisting with perineal care

6. ____ Giving a massage to a resident with acne on his back

7. ____ Hugging residents

8. ____ Shaving a resident

9. List guidelines for handling linen and equipment

Crossword Puzzle

Across

4. Type of container in which sharps should be disposed

5. Linen should be rolled so that the dirtiest area is here

6. Nursing assistants should not do this to dirty linen or clothes

Down

1. Another word for "single-use" equipment

2. Something that must be worn when handling soiled linen

3. Guidelines for the storage and disposal of linens and equipment are set by this government agency.

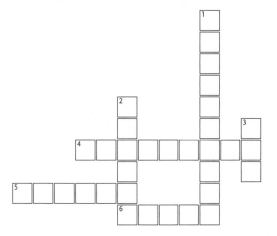

10. Explain how to handle spills

Short Answer

1. Why are spills in a healthcare facility dangerous?

_____

_____

_____

_____

2. When something is spilled, what is the first step that a nursing assistant should take?

_____

_____

_____

_____

3. If a nursing assistant spills a substance on her body, what should she do?

_____

_____

_____

_____

_____

11. Discuss Transmission-Based Precautions

Short Answer
Write the correct type of isolation precaution: "A" for Airborne, "D" for Droplet, or "C" for Contact for each of the following.

1. ____ These are used when the disease-causing microorganism only travels short distances after being expelled.

2. ____ Transmission of a microorganism can occur with direct contact, for example, a nursing assistant bathing a resident.

3. ____ These precautions reduce the risk of spreading tuberculosis.

4. ____ Microorganisms can be spread by talking, singing, sneezing, laughing or coughing.

5. ____ Diseases can be transmitted through the air over long distances.

6. ____ Infection can be spread by touching contaminated personal items.

12. Describe care of the resident in an isolation unit

Short Answer

1. Why is it important to spend as much time as possible with a resident who is in isolation?

_____

_____

_____

_____

2. List five guidelines for residents in isolation that a nursing assistant should follow.

_____

_____

_____

_____

_____

_____

_____

_____

_____

_____

_____

_____

_____

_____

3. What are items that may be needed when setting up an isolation cart?

_____

_____

_____

_____

_____

13. Explain OSHA's Bloodborne Pathogen Standard

Word Search

1. _____ is the abbreviation of the government agency that regulates the safety of workers in the U.S.

2. The _____ Standard is the law that requires healthcare facilities to protect employees from bloodborne health hazards.

3. A(n) _____ is when an employee is exposed to blood or other potentially infectious material.

4. A(n) _____ plan outlines specific work practices to prevent exposure to infectious material and identifies step-by-step procedures to follow when exposures do occur.

5. Infection can be spread by having accidental contact with contaminated blood or body fluids, skin, _____ or other sharp objects, or _____ supplies or equipment.

6. The employer is responsible for providing a free _____ vaccine to all employees after hire.

```
c  i  l  b  f  l  j  t  y  n  k  v  l  h
l  a  o  l  k  o  y  n  b  q  s  a  g  c
m  g  b  o  m  r  c  e  g  z  k  p  h  j
u  w  k  o  q  t  q  d  u  k  m  t  v  m
s  t  v  d  v  n  c  i  o  v  q  j  x  q
g  v  a  b  b  o  q  c  t  a  w  e  o  w
t  k  r  o  i  c  l  n  m  b  k  n  m  x
u  w  b  r  j  e  y  i  y  n  x  s  y  a
o  l  g  n  e  r  y  e  e  b  c  o  k  f
d  s  d  e  t  u  c  r  a  b  k  b  d  h
h  v  h  p  x  s  c  u  z  t  k  s  c  p
c  t  a  a  x  o  a  s  r  w  k  i  a  l
s  s  z  t  w  p  s  o  l  b  n  t  e  d
a  p  a  h  f  x  o  p  g  w  t  i  d  a
b  y  r  o  o  e  h  x  u  h  c  t  c  q
i  m  d  g  w  u  w  e  c  i  o  a  g  g
n  m  s  e  l  d  e  e  n  e  p  p  a  k
j  c  o  n  t  a  m  i  n  a  t  e  d  h
l  b  a  t  e  r  t  d  p  y  s  h  y  a
h  d  u  m  e  t  l  l  z  u  g  p  w  c
```

14. Discuss two important bloodborne diseases

Multiple Choice

1. How does HIV cause the body to be unable to fight infection?
   (A) Causes cirrhosis
   (B) Causes liver cancer
   (C) Damages the immune system
   (D) Poisons the blood

2. What is one way that HIV is spread?
   (A) By coughing or sneezing
   (B) By using infected needles
   (C) By hugging
   (D) Through handshakes

3. Hepatitis ___ and ___ are bloodborne diseases that can cause death.
   (A) A and B
   (B) B and C
   (C) C and E
   (D) A and C

4. Which of the following statements is true of hepatitis B?
   (A) Hepatitis B is commonly spread by the fecal-oral route.
   (B) There is no vaccine for hepatitis B.
   (C) Hepatitis B can be spread by contact with infected needles.
   (D) Hepatitis B can be spread through contaminated water.

15. Discuss MRSA, VRE, and C. *difficile*

True or False

1. ____ Multidrug-resistant organisms (MDROs) are not a serious problem in healthcare facilities.

2. ____ Methicillin-resistant *Staphylococcus aureus* (MRSA) is mostly spread by direct physical contact.

3. ____ The most important way to control MRSA and vancomycin-resistant *enterococcus* (VRE) is through proper hand hygiene.

4. ____ The bacterium *enterococcus* often causes problems in healthy people.

5. ____ VRE is normally easily controlled with the use of antibiotics.

6. ____ Both hand rubs and washing hands with soap and water are considered equally effective when dealing with C. *difficile*.

7. ____ Overuse of antibiotics may alter the normal intestinal flora and increase the risk of developing C. *difficile* diarrhea.

8. ____ There is no test that can diagnose C. *difficile*.

7

Safety and Body Mechanics

1. Review the key terms in Learning Objective 1 before completing the workbook exercises

2. List common accidents in facilities and ways to prevent them

True or False

1. _____ An important way to help prevent falls is to respond to call lights promptly.

2. _____ Wearing long clothing and going without shoes are helpful in preventing falls.

3. _____ A nursing assistant must identify each resident before providing care or serving food.

4. _____ Disoriented or confused residents should not be identified before serving food since they do not understand who they are anyway.

5. _____ Burns can cause a rapid deterioration in a resident's condition.

6. _____ In order to prevent burns, the water temperature should be 130°F when giving a bath.

7. _____ Liquids can cause burns.

8. _____ A disoriented resident may eat hair care products or flowers.

9. _____ To aid in choking prevention, residents should eat quickly.

10. _____ Sitting up straight while eating helps prevent choking.

11. _____ Large pieces of food are less likely to cause choking.

12. _____ Protecting arms and legs while moving residents helps prevent injury.

13. _____ If a nursing assistant needs help lifting a resident, but nobody is around, she should lift the resident anyway.

14. _____ If no eye wash station is available after an eye splash, rinse the eye immediately with water at a sink.

3. Explain the Material Safety Data Sheet (MSDS)

Short Answer

1. List five examples of information that are found on an MSDS.

_____

_____

_____

_____

_____

_____

_____

_____

2. What are two things that a nursing assistant must know about the MSDS?

_____

_____

_____

_____

_____

4. Describe safety guidelines for sharps and biohazard containers

Fill in the Blank

1. Always wear _____ when disposing of infectious waste.

2. It is important to keep _____ above the opening of a biohazard container.

3. When touching a sharps container, touch the _____ of the container only.

4. Sharps containers should be replaced when they are _____ full or following facility policy.

5. Biohazard containers and bags are used to dispose of anything contaminated with infectious waste except for anything _____ .

5. Explain the principles of body mechanics and apply them to daily activities

Matching
Use each letter only once.

1. _____ Back and body injuries

2. _____ Body mechanics

3. _____ Alignment

4. _____ Base of support

5. _____ Center of gravity

(A) Foundation that supports an object

(B) The point in the body where the most weight is concentrated

(C) When the two sides of the body are mirror images of each other

(D) The way the parts of the body work together when a person moves

(E) Important problems that nursing assistants face

Short Answer

1. List five activities in a facility that require moving or lifting something.

_____
_____
_____
_____
_____
_____
_____
_____
_____

2. List eight ways to use proper body mechanics on the job.

_____
_____
_____
_____
_____
_____
_____
_____
_____
_____
_____
_____
_____
_____
_____

6. Define two types of restraints and discuss problems associated with restraints

Multiple Choice

1. Why has the use of restraints in facilities been restricted?
   (A) Restraints are too expensive.
   (B) Restraint usage was abused by caregivers.
   (C) Training nursing assistants to use restraints is too difficult.
   (D) Nursing assistants do not have time to monitor residents who are restrained.

2. When may restraints be used?
   (A) For staff convenience
   (B) With a doctor's order
   (C) To discipline residents
   (D) Whenever staff wants to use them

3. Which of the following is a potential effect of restraint use?
   (A) Pressure ulcers
   (B) Increased blood circulation
   (C) Increased bone mass
   (D) Better sleep habits

7. Define the terms "restraint free" and "restraint alternatives" and list examples of restraint alternatives

Word Search

1. _____
   care means that restraints are not kept or used for any reason.

2. Creative ideas that help avoid the use of restraints are called _____
   _____.

3. Answer _____
   _____
   immediately.

4. Add more _____
   into the care plan.

5. Let confused residents
   _____
   in designated safe areas.

6. Increase visits and _____
   interaction.

7. Increase number of familiar
   _____.

8. Decrease the _____
   level.

9. Use soothing _____.

10. Bed or body _____
    alert staff when residents attempt to leave the bed or chair.

```
i s p h v r a z c d f c x b
c e x k d o v v k c f a c q
t v o h t p w a n d e r p q
i i d r v t c e h z u e f a
k t c x l y g j s n o g i c
r a q a r i o x m u s i c k
d n m h d t o n e l y v z c
d r d s a k h o d a q e k r
s e p k m p m g r e j r e v
n t d o x r n p r x d s n v
t l e b m b a x g e t d m s
t a d s l f i l n r e u n j
s t h g i l l l a c p s k x
o n o c m o c i c i b g h j
y i r y z r n q t s c v r n
v a q h t t f j q e l o x g
s r l s f p k j b m h f s g
x t f r a o d i s j b m n n
k s e o f l k x h p s b x v
i e p e n w k w p i y s x f
j r r p r p h d g u i g i d
```

8. Identify what must be done if a restraint is ordered

Crossword Puzzle

Across

2. The medical term for skin that is blue-tinged, gray, or pale

4. Restraints should never be tied to these

5. Before a restraint is applied, the nursing assistant must make sure there is one of these

Down

1. Position in which the hand should be placed between the resident and the restraint to ensure that the device fits properly and is comfortable

2. Way for residents to call for help when they are restrained

3. Type of knot that should be used to tie restraints

6. Restraints must be released at least every _____ hours

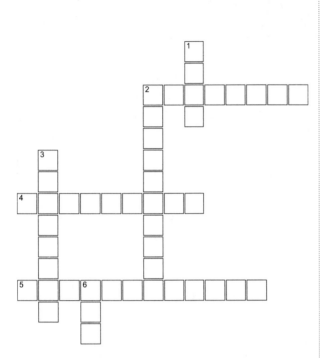

9. List safety guidelines for oxygen use

True or False

1. ____ Nursing assistants should adjust oxygen levels if they seem low.

2. ____ Oxygen is a dangerous fire hazard.

3. ____ Smoking should not be allowed anywhere around oxygen equipment.

4. ____ Fire hazards that should be removed from residents' rooms include electric razors and hair dryers.

5. ____ Combustion means that something is full and ready to burst.

6. ____ The use of lighters and matches is allowed around oxygen.

7. ____ Alcohol and nail polish remover are considered flammable liquids.

8. ____ Oxygen tubing should remain lying flat underneath the resident at all times.

10. Identify safety guidelines for intravenous (IV) lines

Fill in the Blank

1. "IV" is an abbreviation for _____, or into a vein.

2. A resident with an IV is receiving _____, nutrition, or _____ through a vein.

3. A nursing assistant should always wear _____ if she has to touch the IV area.

4. Do not take resident's _____ _____ in an arm with an IV.

5. Do not leave the tubing _____.

6. Do not disconnect the IV from the _____ or turn off the _____.

7. Report to the nurse if the needle or _____ has fallen out.

8. Report to the nurse if _____ appears in the tubing.

9. Report if the resident complains of _____ or has difficulty _____.

10. Residents who have IVs have the right to freedom of _____.

11. Discuss fire safety and explain the "RACE" and "PASS" acronyms

Short Answer

1. What are the three things needed for a fire to occur?

_____

_____

_____

_____

_____

2. List five potential causes of fire in facilities.

_____

_____

_____

_____

_____

_____

_____

3. Fill in the words for the following acronyms:

R _____

A _____

C _____

E _____

P _____

A _____

S _____

S _____

4. List four general procedures to follow in case of a fire.

_____

_____

_____

_____

_____

_____

_____

12. List general safety steps to protect yourself and residents in a facility

True or False

1. _____ Living or working in a facility means a person is safe from all crime.

2. _____ Very few people go in and out of a facility during the day.

3. _____ It is best to watch for suspicious behavior and report it immediately.

4. _____ It is a good idea for a nursing assistant to take valuables to work so that he can keep an eye on them.

5. _____ A nursing assistant should not leave a resident alone with a visitor or staff member who makes her uneasy.

6. _____ Personal information about residents and staff may be shared with anyone who asks.

Name: _____

8

Emergency Care, First Aid, and Disasters

1. Review the key terms in Learning Objective 1 before completing the workbook exercises

2. Demonstrate how to respond to medical emergencies

Short Answer

1. When a nursing assistant is assessing an emergency situation, what should he or she do?

_____

_____

_____

2. When a nursing assistant is assessing a victim in a medical emergency, what should he or she do?

_____

_____

_____

_____

_____

_____

_____

_____

_____

3. Demonstrate knowledge of first aid procedures

Word Search

1. When breathing stops, it is called

_____

arrest.

2. When the heart stops, it is called

_____

arrest.

3. _____

_____

refers to medical procedures used when the heart or lungs have stopped working; it is used until medical help arrives.

4. CPR must be started immediately to prevent or minimize

_____.

5. Brain damage can occur within _____ to _____ minutes after breathing stops and the heart stops beating.

6. Only properly _____ people should perform CPR.

7. _____

is the care given by the first people to respond to an emergency.

Name: _____

```
r t x c j f l g j l i b l t
c c v a m l p a h h j v r a
z x u r v g h p t t i d l a
u d o d q h u g q y x z k e
e l h i y v x d c i p b p b
o t w o q e g n e b r g y b
g k o p f z c v r a c u b z
j s i u b t a d i q j h o e
v g r l c a i n z r w k z f
l o v m o s d z x k w o u o
w y r o t a r i p s e r j i
z f v n m j a d d y t l v p
n i o a l d c i g h n p c s
b n g r u i j i e i e v g y
g e z y w d z r d o q z a q
t c q r f z i q o w u y l c
v c p e f n a x z d q j j l
c r w s x e j n e f j f x o
f l m u q a f n o g v z d f
f i r s t a i d y z i d y t
t x w c z a g o w d q h c b
c n a i r b b a t h l a s c
l x g t u p l w w r y g g b
e m a a x r c c e l b e n c
j t o t t g v h d v h s p i
i d s i x a l a d a q c i l
s c y o a v o b g q v p v n
r b w n j k e t l i y x o f
```

True or False

1. ____ Normally when a person is choking, she lies face down on the ground.

2. ____ The nursing assistant should leave the choking victim alone in order to find someone to help her.

3. ____ Before giving abdominal thrusts, the nursing assistant should ask the victim if he or she is choking.

4. ____ A person in shock should sit upright until symptoms improve.

5. ____ After notifying the nurse, the first step a nursing assistant should take when trying to control bleeding is to put on gloves.

6. ____ When blood seeps through a pad that is being used to control bleeding, it should be removed and replaced with a clean pad.

7. ____ Applying butter or cooking oil to a serious burn will help reduce the chance of infection.

8. ____ If a person appears likely to faint and is sitting down, the nursing assistant should have her bend forward and put her head between her knees.

9. ____ The medical term for vomiting is epistaxis.

10. ____ When a person has vomited, it is important to check vomitus for blood or medication.

11. ____ Men are more likely than women to deny that they are having a heart attack.

12. ____ If a nursing assistant suspects a person is having a heart attack, she should give him water right away.

13. ____ The medical term for a heart attack is transient ischemic attack (TIA).

14. ____ Insulin reaction results from too much insulin or too little food.

15. ____ Diabetic ketoacidosis may be caused by undiagnosed diabetes.

16. ____ If a resident is having a seizure, the nursing assistant should put his fingers in the resident's mouth so that the resident will be able to breathe.

17. ____ The response time to a suspected stroke is important, as early treatment can reduce severity of the stroke.

18. ____ Slurring of words and facial droop are two important signs to report that may signal a stroke is beginning.

Matching

For each sign or symptom or response described below, write the letter of the medical emergency it applies to. Use each letter only once.

1. ____ Signs of this include pale or cyanotic skin, staring, increased pulse and respiration rates, decreased blood pressure, and extreme thirst.

2. ____ Hold a thick sterile pad directly against the wound.

3. ____ Signs of this include severe pain in the chest, anxiety, and heartburn or indigestion.

4. ____ Performing abdominal thrusts may help with this emergency.

5. ____ Apply firm pressure over the bridge of the nose if this occurs.

6. ____ Never use any kind of ointment, water, salve, or grease on this.

7. ____ If a person is sitting, have her bend forward and place her head between her knees.

8. ____ Signs of this include use of strange words, loss of bowel and bladder control, and blurred vision.

9. ____ Do not try to stop this or hold the person down.

10. ____ Sweet or fruity breath is a symptom.

11. ____ If this occurs, it is a good idea to give the person a lump of sugar, candy, or a glass of orange juice immediately.

12. ____ Giving oral care after this happens is helpful.

13. ____ Signs of this include sudden collapse, vomiting, and heavy, difficult breathing.

(A) Bleeding

(B) Burn

(C) Choking

(D) Diabetic ketoacidosis (hyperglycemia)

(E) Fainting (syncope)

(F) Insulin reaction (hypoglycemia)

(G) Myocardial infarction

(H) Nosebleed (epistaxis)

(I) Poisoning

(J) Seizure

(K) Shock

(L) Stroke

(M) Vomiting (emesis)

4. Explain the nursing assistant's role on a code team

Fill in the Blank

1. Facilities use codes to inform staff of

_____

without alarming residents and visitors.

2. "Code Red" usually means

_____,

and "Code Blue" usually means

_____.

3. The _____
is the team chosen for a shift to respond in case of a resident emergency.

4. Staff on the code team may be asked to get a special _____
or other emergency equipment.

5. Nursing assistants may be asked to do

_____

during CPR.

6. Respond to codes after any residents you are caring for are _____.

5. Describe guidelines for responding to disasters

Short Answer

1. What kinds of disasters are most likely to occur in your area?

_____

_____

_____

_____

_____

_____

_____

2. Describe the way nursing assistants should respond to disasters.

_____

_____

_____

_____

_____

_____

_____

_____

9

Admission, Transfer, Discharge, and Physical Exams

1. Review the key terms in Learning Objective 1 before completing the workbook exercises

2. List factors for families in choosing a facility

Short Answer

1. What are three sources of information that families may use to guide them in choosing a facility for a loved one?

_____

_____

_____

_____

_____

2. Why do you think family members ask so many questions before deciding on a facility for their loved one?

_____

_____

_____

_____

_____

_____

3. Explain the nursing assistant's role in the emotional adjustment of a new resident

Scenario
Read the following scenario and answer the questions that follow.

New resident Isabelle Marks is having a hard time. She mostly cries in her room and refuses to participate in any activity. Nursing assistant Tyson Chandler stops by her room to take her blood pressure. When he sees her crying by the window, he sighs loudly and rolls his eyes. "You're lucky I'm here," he says. "Nobody else knows how to deal with emotional residents."

He continues, "In fact, last week the resident in room 102 couldn't stop crying when he found out he has colon cancer. I was the only one he would talk to."

Ms. Marks continues to cry softly while he takes her blood pressure. "I don't know why you're so sad," he says. "I'd be happy if I could be somewhere where I got all my meals cooked and my room cleaned. Plus, there's lots of other old folks here to talk to."

He leaves her room and realizes he forgot to note her blood pressure. Not wanting to deal with her again, he thinks for a moment and writes down some numbers.

1. Name seven things Tyson could have done to take better care of Ms. Marks.

_____

_____

_____

Name: _____

_____
_____
_____
_____
_____
_____
_____
_____
_____
_____
_____
_____

2. List five reasons that moving into a facility is a big emotional adjustment for new residents.

_____
_____
_____
_____
_____
_____
_____
_____
_____
_____

4. Describe the nursing assistant's role in the admission process

True or False

1. ____ In order to keep a new resident occupied, let him or her figure out how to use the bed controls and the call light.

2. ____ Family and friends are a good source of information for a resident's personal preferences, history, and routines.

3. ____ A new resident's admission pack may include soap, a bedpan, a pitcher, and a cup.

4. ____ It is better to wait until the resident has already arrived to start preparing her room.

5. ____ The resident should not feel as if he is an inconvenience; he should feel welcome and wanted.

6. ____ It is important to introduce new residents to other residents and staff members.

7. ____ Baseline measurements are taken six months after admission to a facility.

8. ____ Changes in residents' weight do not need to be reported.

9. ____ Residents who cannot get out of bed cannot have their height or weight measured.

10. ____ When measuring height, remember that there are eight inches in a foot.

5. Explain the nursing assistant's role during an in-house transfer of a resident

Word Search

1. Residents may need to be transferred to a unit that offers more _____ care.

2. _____ is always hard. This may be especially true if the resident has a(n) _____ or his condition has _____.

3. Nursing assistants should try to make the transfer as _____ as possible for residents.

4. Residents have the right to be _____ of any room or roommate change.

5. At the new unit, _____ the resident to everyone.

6. If a nursing assistant _____ the resident's belongings, she should do it carefully.

7. When leaving the resident's room, report to the _____ in charge of the resident.

```
p  l  i  f  s  w  t  x  b  w  f  k  y  g
z  s  c  r  m  n  e  u  p  i  f  a  a  b
e  u  h  s  y  t  c  c  q  h  t  d  n  f
c  r  a  k  o  y  u  p  t  j  e  e  r  n
h  p  n  c  o  u  d  o  n  i  b  l  i  m
g  d  g  a  s  t  o  u  f  r  g  l  o  i
e  r  e  p  s  m  r  i  x  j  b  i  e  r
y  n  u  n  s  s  t  c  f  k  c  k  s  i
n  z  s  u  e  o  n  t  x  t  t  s  g  b
i  x  t  v  n  s  i  v  x  e  b  n  a  h
b  u  l  m  l  e  r  r  p  x  m  y  e  e
x  l  u  h  l  v  e  o  m  a  m  s  m  l
k  x  j  n  i  a  r  l  w  j  s  g  d  i
y  l  a  o  v  j  u  u  r  i  p  k  a  z
```

6. Explain the nursing assistant's role in the discharge of a resident

Multiple Choice

1. When does a resident's discharge from the facility become official?
   (A) After the doctor writes the discharge order that releases the resident to leave the facility
   (B) After the resident is informed of the discharge
   (C) After the resident leaves the facility
   (D) When the nurse gives the resident instructions to be followed after discharge

2. Which of the following is the nursing assistant's responsibility during discharge?
   (A) Collecting and packing the resident's belongings
   (B) Giving the resident any special dietary instructions
   (C) Writing the discharge order
   (D) Reviewing medications that the resident needs to take

3. A nursing assistant is responsible for the resident until:
   (A) The discharge order has been written by the doctor.
   (B) The resident's items are packed, and the inventory list has been checked.
   (C) The resident is outside the facility.
   (D) The resident is safely in the vehicle with the doors closed.

Short Answer

1. Explain what it means when a resident leaves a facility "AMA."

   _____
   _____
   _____
   _____
   _____
   _____
   _____
   _____

2. What happens when a resident wants to leave AMA?

   _____
   _____
   _____
   _____
   _____
   _____

7. Describe the nursing assistant's role during physical exams

Multiple Choice

1. What are the nursing assistant's duties during residents' physical exams?
   (A) Performing the exams
   (B) Giving injections
   (C) Diagnosing illness or disease
   (D) Getting equipment for the doctor or nurse

2. In which position is the resident placed for examination of the breasts, chest, abdomen, and perineal area?
   (A) Dorsal recumbent
   (B) Lithotomy position
   (C) Knee-chest position
   (D) Trendelenburg position

3. Which of the following pieces of equipment is used to measure blood pressure?
   (A) Reflex hammer
   (B) Thermometer
   (C) Sphygmomanometer
   (D) Otoscope

4. In which position is the resident in stirrups in order to examine the vagina?
   (A) Sims' position
   (B) Lithotomy position
   (C) Knee-chest position
   (D) Prone position

5. Which position is used to examine the rectum or the vagina?
   (A) Lateral position
   (B) Lithotomy position
   (C) Knee-chest position
   (D) Prone position

10

Bedmaking and Unit Care

1. Review the key terms in Learning Objective 1 before completing the workbook exercises

2. Discuss the importance of sleep

Fill in the Blank

1. _____ is a natural period of rest for the mind and body during which _____ is restored.

2. Sleep is needed to replace old _____ with new ones and provide new energy to _____.

3. Deep sleep helps the body to _____.

4. _____ are natural rhythms and cycles related to body functions.

5. The _____ _____ is the 24-hour day-night cycle.

3. Describe types of sleep disorders

Matching
Use each letter only once.

1. _____ REM sleep behavior disorder

2. _____ Insomnia

3. _____ Sleeptalking

4. _____ Parasomnias

5. _____ Somnambulism

6. _____ Bruxism

(A) Talking during sleep

(B) Grinding and clenching the teeth

(C) Sleepwalking

(D) Inability to fall asleep or to remain asleep

(E) Sleep disorders

(F) Talking, often along with violent movements, during REM sleep

4. Identify factors affecting sleep

Scenario
Read the following scenario and answer the questions that follow.

New resident Anne Ross has been having trouble sleeping. She generally has dinner, dessert, and coffee around 8:30 p.m. every day. Her husband recently died in the home they shared together for 24 years. After his death, she started a new medication to help with her depression. Her roommate, Riva, likes to sleep with the light on because she frequently has to use the bathroom. Sometimes Riva is unable to make it to the bathroom in time and has to call a nursing assistant for help. The nursing assistant will change the sheets and help Riva clean herself as quickly as possible.

1. List five factors that could be affecting Anne's ability to sleep.

_____

_____

_____

_____

_____

_____

Name: _____

_____

_____

_____

2. For each factor you listed above, suggest a solution that might help Anne sleep better.

_____

_____

_____

_____

_____

_____

_____

_____

_____

3. List four problems that can be caused by not sleeping well.

_____

_____

_____

_____

_____

_____

_____

5. Describe a standard resident unit and equipment

Short Answer

For each of the following, Make a check mark (✓) beside the standard equipment you will see in most resident units.

1. ____ Overbed table

2. ____ Mechanical lift

3. ____ Call light

4. ____ Children

5. ____ Bed

6. ____ Bedpan

7. ____ Massage table

8. ____ Emesis basin

True or False

1. ____ A nursing assistant must always knock and wait for permission before entering a resident's room.

2. ____ Residents' personal items are not very important to them.

3. ____ If a safety hazard exists in a resident's room, the nursing assistant should remove it immediately.

4. ____ Personal articles can be stored in the bedside stand.

5. ____ Bedpans should be stored on overbed tables.

6. ____ When making a bed, the nursing assistant should place soiled linen on the overbed table.

6. Explain how to clean a resident unit and equipment

Multiple Choice

1. General care of the resident's unit must be done:
   (A) Once a day
   (B) Whenever it is needed throughout the day
   (C) Once a week
   (D) Only when the resident asks

2. Which of the following is an example of disposable equipment?
   (A) Bedpan
   (B) Stethoscope
   (C) Gloves
   (D) Blood pressure cuff

3. The call light must always be kept:
    (A) Within the resident's reach
    (B) Near the door
    (C) On the bedside stand
    (D) On the overbed table

4. Which of the following duties is the nursing assistant responsible for with regard to cleaning a resident's unit after he is transferred, discharged, or dies?
    (A) Notifying people on the facility's waiting list that a room is ready
    (B) Removing equipment and supplies
    (C) Throwing away any of the resident's remaining personal items
    (D) Repairing damaged or broken furniture

7. Discuss types of beds and demonstrate proper bedmaking

True or False

1. _____ Some beds have built-in scales for weighing bedridden residents.

2. _____ Wrinkles, soiled linens, and lumps in beds can cause pressure ulcers and must be avoided.

3. _____ A nursing assistant should wear gloves when removing soiled linens.

4. _____ Clean linen should be carried away from a nursing assistant's uniform.

5. _____ Linen can be transferred from one resident's room to another resident's room.

6. _____ Bed linen should be shaken to clean it of any microorganisms.

7. _____ An open bed is made for a resident who will be out of bed all day.

8. _____ It is easier to make an occupied bed than an unoccupied bed.

9. _____ A nursing assistant should roll dirty linen away from her as it is removed from the bed.

10. _____ Using proper body mechanics when making a bed means that the nursing assistant should keep her knees straight and her feet close together.

11

Positioning, Moving, and Lifting

1. Review the key terms in Learning Objective 1 before completing the workbook exercises

2. Explain body alignment and review the principles of body mechanics

Word Search

1. _____ the load.

2. Think ahead, _____ and communicate the move.

3. Check base of _____ and be sure to have firm

_____,

4. _____ what you are lifting.

5. Keep back _____.

6. Begin in a squatting position and lift with the _____.

7. _____ stomach muscles when beginning the lift.

8. Keep the object _____ to the body.

9. Do not _____, as it increases stress on the back.

10. _____ when possible rather than lifting.

```
s  y  s  s  o  l  r  q  s  o  u  h  z  l
o  t  r  o  p  p  u  s  h  a  u  y  n  c
f  e  r  i  l  d  q  m  f  o  o  l  i  m
a  j  u  a  o  t  w  z  p  k  q  e  d  x
f  n  n  i  i  i  m  f  q  w  f  h  q  d
m  n  a  f  t  g  s  w  f  o  w  f  b  r
j  b  k  s  d  h  h  u  o  q  j  m  n  p
o  t  w  i  s  t  c  t  k  c  z  h  p  j
m  w  u  n  l  e  i  b  e  l  r  t  j  e
q  s  e  s  h  n  s  e  b  g  k  x  i  i
q  j  v  w  g  s  y  s  c  p  u  e  k  v
v  v  d  u  w  e  i  o  b  w  d  e  t  h
r  p  p  r  x  u  l  l  z  l  c  h  y  i
o  e  c  y  t  p  e  c  a  f  a  w  e  z
```

3. Explain why position changes are important for bedbound residents and describe basic body positions

Matching
Use each letter only once.

1. ____ Dangling

2. ____ Draw sheet

3. ____ Fowler's

4. ____ Lateral

5. ____ Logrolling

6. ____ Positioning

7. ____ Prone

8. ____ Reverse Trendelenburg

Name: _____

9. ____ Shearing

10. ____ Sims'

11. ____ Supine

12. ____ Trendelenburg

(A) Semi-sitting position (45 to 60 degrees)

(B) An extra sheet placed on top of the bottom sheet to help prevent skin damage caused by shearing

(C) Helping residents into positions that promote comfort and good health

(D) Position in which resident is lying on his or her stomach

(E) Position that may be used for a resident who needs a faster emptying of the stomach due to a digestive problem

(F) Sitting up with the legs hanging over the side of the bed to regain balance

(G) Position in which a resident is lying on either side

(H) Left side-lying position in which the upper knee is flexed and raised toward the chest

(I) Position in which the resident is lying flat on his back

(J) Rubbing or friction resulting from the skin moving one way and the bone underneath it remaining fixed or moving in the opposite direction

(K) Position that may be used for a resident who has gone into shock and has poor blood flow

(L) Method of moving a resident as a unit, without disturbing the alignment of the body

Short Answer

1. Why is it important to reposition and turn bedbound residents often?

_____

_____

_____

_____

_____

_____

_____

_____

_____

2. List three things that a nursing assistant should check a resident's skin for each time a resident is repositioned.

_____

_____

_____

_____

_____

_____

_____

_____

4. Describe how to safely transfer residents

Multiple Choice

1. How should a nursing assistant transfer a resident who has a strong side and a weak side?
   (A) The weaker side moves first.
   (B) The strong side moves first.
   (C) Both sides must move together at the same time.
   (D) It does not matter which side moves first.

2. The science of designing equipment, areas, and tasks to make them safer and to suit the worker's abilities is called:
   (A) Musculoskeletal motion
   (B) Oncology
   (C) Ergonomics
   (D) Biology

3. Which of the following is a proper guideline for resident transfers?
   (A) Whenever the nursing assistant can, she should manually lift the resident to move him from one place to another.
   (B) Having a "zero lift" policy in place means that a nursing assistant should be able to lift the resident on her own, without help.
   (C) Safety is not as much of a concern during transferring a resident as it is while positioning a resident.
   (D) It is important for the nursing assistant to get the help she needs when lifting a resident.

4. Which of the following is true of transfer belts?
   (A) They are called slide belts when used to help residents walk.
   (B) They are used most often for residents with fragile bones or recent fractures.
   (C) They fit around the resident's waist, over his clothes.
   (D) They are the same as mechanical lifts.

5. Sliding boards are used for:
   (A) Transferring residents who cannot bear weight on their legs from one sitting position to another
   (B) Helping weak residents ambulate for longer distances
   (C) Easier lifting of residents who can only bear weight on one leg
   (D) Transferring weak residents who are standing to a sitting position

6. Which of the following is true of using a wheelchair?
   (A) A resident's hips should be positioned at the very front of the chair.
   (B) When moving down a ramp, go down forward, with the resident facing the bottom of the ramp.
   (C) When using an elevator, turn the chair around so that the resident faces forward.
   (D) The wheels of the wheelchair should be unlocked while the nursing assistant is positioning a resident.

7. Which of the following is true of mechanical lifts?
   (A) Mechanical lifts help protect staff and residents from injury during lifting.
   (B) Mechanical lifts are commonly used to transfer residents into ambulances.
   (C) Mechanical lifts are often used in place of wheelchairs as a way for residents to move around the facility.
   (D) Mechanical lifts are used in the dining room to help with safe food service.

8. For a resident to be able to use a toilet, he must be able to:
   (A) Walk to the toilet without assistance
   (B) Stand up without assistance
   (C) Bear some weight on his legs
   (D) Transfer himself from a wheelchair to the toilet without assistance

5. Discuss ambulation

Multiple Choice

1. Ambulation is another term for:
   (A) Emergency care
   (B) Riding
   (C) Dangling
   (D) Walking

2. Before assisting a resident to ambulate, his or her feet should be
   (A) Flat on the floor
   (B) Pointed to the side
   (C) Pointed upward
   (D) Barefoot

3. When helping a visually-impaired resident walk, the nursing assistant should:
   (A) Make sure the gait belt is directly over the resident's bare skin
   (B) Walk slightly behind the resident
   (C) Walk slightly in front of the resident
   (D) Remain about 12 inches apart from the resident's side

12

Personal Care

1. Review the key terms in Learning Objective 1 before completing the workbook exercises

2. Explain personal care of residents

True or False

1. _____ Good grooming helps keep a person clean and healthy.

2. _____ The nursing assistant will make all the decisions about how to groom a resident.

3. _____ All residents will be bathed in the morning after they wake up.

4. _____ The nursing assistant should insist that residents brush their teeth before eating breakfast.

5. _____ *Grooming* is the term to describe methods of keeping the body clean, while *hygiene* includes practices like fingernail, foot, and hair care.

6. _____ Helping residents with their activities of daily living (ADLs) is outside of a nursing assistant's scope of practice.

7. _____ The nursing assistant should perform as much personal care as possible for the resident so that the resident does not become frustrated.

8. _____ Residents may be embarrassed by having someone else provide personal care.

9. _____ Residents have the right to choose what they want to wear, including jewelry.

10. _____ Residents should be left alone during bathing to promote independence.

11. _____ The nursing assistant should let the resident know that he is only allowed to use the toilet for a few minutes.

12. _____ The nursing assistant should keep residents covered as much as possible when bathing and dressing them.

3. Describe different types of baths and list observations to make about the skin during bathing

Short Answer

1. List the four basic types of baths. For each one, list one type of resident for which this bath is best suited.

_____

_____

_____

_____

_____

_____

_____

_____

_____

_____

_____

_____

2. How is the decision made about which kind of bath a resident will receive?

_____

_____

_____

_____

_____

_____

3. List ten things to observe and report during personal care and bathing.

_____

_____

_____

_____

_____

_____

_____

_____

_____

_____

_____

_____

4. Explain safety guidelines for bathing

Word Search

1. A nursing assistant should not try to

   _____

   a resident alone if he does not believe he can handle the task.

2. Make sure the floor in the shower or tub room is _____. Wipe up any _____ or wet areas.

3. Place _____ mats in regular tubs.

4. Check to see that _____ and _____ are secure and in proper working order.

5. Bath _____, _____, and powder can create slippery surfaces and can put residents at risk of falling.

6. Check water temperature with a

   _____

   or on the wrist.

7. Do not use _____

   _____ near a water

   source.

```
n m e c t s w c b j y t l w
f s l i a r d n a h s f t g
s h e h t a b s t d d y f j
m g c k s b r c h v t s c t
i g t d l b u e t i b t x c
f n r q e a g v h m d q j g
e y i z g r h d e b d a b b
h k c o y g x n r i l p e c
e n a f m v p v m d o g i e
e m l t x d g p o z c a p e
j c a z n f z i m x a j x s
h m p b a o k i e k a d x i
h s p l z l e k t m a r o g
l j l w n e r k e m t y y d
c p i l s n o n r e x p b m
o h a k i m i n r t f k e y
x w n h o p l o q x w f f c
w t c i x n s a z k k c v j
q o e g o r q m x a x f l l
r z s w a p q c e f y b y d
```

5. List the order in which body parts are washed during bathing

Short Answer

1. Why is it important to follow a specific order when bathing a person?

_____

_____

_____

_____

2. State the general rule of the order of parts for bathing.

_____

_____

_____

_____

Labeling

Look at the figure below. In the blanks provided, number the parts of the body in the order in which they should be bathed.

Eyes _____   Neck _____   Face _____

Chest and   Ears _____
abdomen _____

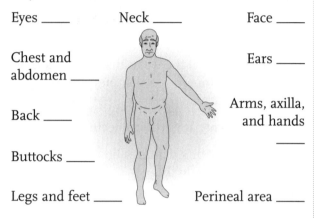

Back _____   Arms, axilla,
                                            and hands

                                            _____

Buttocks _____

Legs and feet _____   Perineal area _____

6. Explain how to assist with bathing

Multiple Choice

1. What opportunity does bathing a resident give the nursing assistant?
   (A) It allows the nursing assistant to talk to other nursing assistants.
   (B) It allows the nursing assistant to see if the resident needs to change her medications.
   (C) It allows the nursing assistant to observe the skin and report changes.
   (D) It allows the nursing assistant to understand how the resident feels about hygiene.

2. Which one of the following parts of the body should be washed every day?
   (A) Hair
   (B) Thighs
   (C) Back
   (D) Perineal area

3. When is a partial bath performed?
   (A) Every day
   (B) Only for testing purposes
   (C) On days when a complete bed bath, tub bath, or shower is not done
   (D) When a resident cannot get out of bed

4. To shampoo hair for a resident on a stretcher, the nursing assistant should:
   (A) Transfer the resident to a bed
   (B) Transfer the resident to a chair in front of the sink
   (C) Bring the stretcher to the sink and adjust the height of the stretcher
   (D) A resident on a stretcher cannot have his hair shampooed.

5. What kind of equipment is used to help a resident into a whirlpool bath?
   (A) Gait belt
   (B) Sliding board
   (C) Chair lift
   (D) Wheelchair

7. Describe how to perform a back rub

True or False

1. _____ It is inappropriate for a nursing assistant to give a resident a back rub.

2. _____ Back rubs help relax muscles and improve circulation.

3. _____ Back rubs need to be given to all residents.

4. _____ The position that is most comfortable for elderly people is lying on their stomachs (prone).

5. _____ Red areas over bony parts of the body should be massaged using long, smooth strokes.

8. Explain guidelines for performing good oral care

Matching
Use each letter only once.

1. _____ Edentulous

2. _____ Gingivitis

Name: _____

3. ____ Halitosis

4. ____ Plaque

5. ____ Tartar

(A) Inflammation of the gums

(B) Substance that accumulates on the teeth from food and bacteria

(C) Bad-smelling breath

(D) Hard deposits on teeth that are filled with bacteria and may cause gum disease and loose teeth

(E) Lacking teeth

Short Answer

1. List seven signs and symptoms to report during oral care.

_____

_____

_____

_____

_____

_____

_____

_____

_____

2. List five ways that a nursing assistant will assist a resident who can brush his own teeth.

_____

_____

_____

_____

_____

_____

_____

_____

_____

9. Define "dentures" and explain care guidelines

Crossword Puzzle

Across

1. A labeled one of these is used to store dentures

5. Temperature of the water that dentures must always be stored in so that they do not dry out and warp

7. Another word for artificial teeth

8. When a person's dentures break, he or she can no longer do this

Down

2. Dentures that are left uncovered can warp, dry out, or do this

3. Must be worn when cleaning dentures

4. A type of dental appliance that replaces missing or pulled teeth

6. Temperature of water that can warp dentures

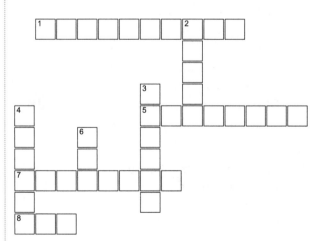

10. Discuss guidelines for performing oral care for an unconscious resident

Multiple Choice

1. Oral care needs to be done frequently for residents who are unconscious for which of the following reasons?
   (A) Too much moisture collects in the mouth
   (B) To encourage the growth of "good" bacteria in the mouth
   (C) The mouth becomes dry due to lack of oral fluids, breathing through the mouth, and oxygen therapy.
   (D) To help make it easier to chew food

2. Aspiration is:
   (A) A crust that appears on the lips, gums, and teeth of people who are unconscious
   (B) A cause of unconsciousness
   (C) Inhalation of food, fluid, or foreign material into the lungs
   (D) A procedure used to create an artificial airway

3. One way to prevent aspiration is to:
   (A) Turn unconscious residents on their backs before beginning oral care
   (B) Avoid performing oral care on unconscious residents
   (C) Use as little liquid as possible during oral care
   (D) Use swabs soaked in large amounts of fluid to clean the mouth

4. Residents who are unconscious may still be able to:
   (A) Hear
   (B) Dress themselves
   (C) Ambulate
   (D) Feed themselves

5. Which of the following statements is true of performing eye care for an unconscious resident?
   (A) The nursing assistant should use gloves when bathing the eye.
   (B) The nursing assistant should wipe from the outer area to the inner area of the eye when cleaning.
   (C) The nursing assistant should use the same cotton ball to clean both eyes.
   (D) The nursing assistant should not speak to an unconscious resident while performing care.

11. Explain how to assist with grooming

True or False

1. _____ Appearance has very little to do with how people feel about themselves.

2. _____ The nursing assistant will make all the decisions about how to groom a resident.

3. _____ A nursing assistant must always wear gloves when shaving residents.

4. _____ All residents need to be shaved.

5. _____ Disposable shaving products should be discarded in the biohazard container.

6. _____ A safety razor is the safest and easiest razor to use.

7. _____ Fingernails can collect and harbor microorganisms.

8. _____ A nursing assistant should cut residents' toenails regularly to keep them healthy.

9. _____ When a resident's hair gets too long, the nursing assistant should trim it.

10. _____ Hair typically thins as a person ages.

11. _____ A nursing assistant should style a resident's in the same style as a little kid's hair is styled; for example, put it in two high ponytails.

12. _____ Lice do not typically spread very quickly.

13. ____ Most residents who have roommates will share their combs and brushes with each other.

14. ____ If a resident has one side of the body that is weaker than the other, it should be referred to as the "affected" or "involved" side.

15. ____ When dressing a resident with one strong side and one weak side, always begin with the strong side.

16. ____ To promote comfort, residents should wear pajamas all day long.

17. ____ Bras that fasten in the back are easier for female residents to manage by themselves.

18. ____ When helping a resident undress, the nursing assistant should begin with the stronger side.

13

Vital Signs

1. Review the key terms in Learning Objective 1 before completing the workbook exercises

2. Discuss the relationship of vital signs to health and well-being

Matching

Match each range with the appropriate vital sign.

1. _____ Oral temperature

2. _____ Normal blood pressure

3. _____ Rectal temperature

4. _____ High blood pressure/hypertension

5. _____ Low blood pressure/hypotension

6. _____ Pulse rate

7. _____ Respiration rate

8. _____ Axillary temperature

9. _____ Prehypertensive

(A) 100/60 – 119/79

(B) 97.6° F – 99.6° F

(C) 120/80 – 139/89

(D) 140/90 or above

(E) 60 – 100 per minute

(F) 12 – 20 per minute

(G) 98.6° F – 100.6° F

(H) 96.6° – 98.6° F

(I) 100/60 or lower

Short Answer

1. List the five vital signs.

_____

_____
_____
_____
_____
_____
_____

2. Why is it important to report changes in vital signs to the nurse?

_____

_____

_____

_____

_____

3. Identify factors that affect body temperature

Multiple Choice

1. Which of the following is the average temperature of the body?
   (A) 98.6° F
   (B) 96.6° F
   (C) 94.8° F
   (D) 99.6° F

2. Severe sub-normal body temperature is called:
   (A) Circadian rhythm
   (B) Hypothalamus
   (C) Hypothermia
   (D) Fever

3. How does a person's age affect body temperature?
   (A) An older person has lost protective fatty tissue, which may cause him or her to feel colder.
   (B) Skin thickens as a person ages, causing him or her to feel warmer.
   (C) An older person no longer exercises, which makes him or her feel colder.
   (D) An older person is ill most of the time, which means he or she feels hot.

4. List guidelines for taking body temperature

Short Answer
Mark an "X" by each person for whom an oral temperature should NOT be taken.

1. _____ Person is confused or disoriented.

2. _____ Person has sores and swelling in his mouth.

3. _____ Person is 40 years old.

4. _____ Person is unconscious.

5. _____ Person has a broken leg.

6. _____ Person is likely to have a seizure.

7. _____ Person has a nasogastric tube.

8. _____ Person has had children.

Short Answer
For each statement below, write an "O" if it refers to oral temperature, an "R" for rectal temperature, a "T" for tympanic temperature, an "A" for axillary temperature, or "TA" for temporal artery.

1. _____ The most common site for taking temperature

2. _____ Thermometer is usually color-coded red

3. _____ Thermometer is lubricated

4. _____ Non-invasive method of measuring temperature

5. _____ May be necessary for unconscious residents

6. _____ Thermometer is inserted only ¼ to ½ inch

7. _____ Site for taking temperature is the armpit

8. _____ Considered to be most accurate

9. _____ Ear wax may cause an inaccurate reading

10. _____ Thermometer is inserted no more than one inch

11. _____ Thermometer is usually color-coded green or blue

12. _____ Probe is moved straight across the forehead

13. _____ Site for taking temperature is the ear

14. _____ Ear injury is possible

Labeling
For each of the mercury-free thermometers shown below, write the temperature reading to the nearest tenth degree.

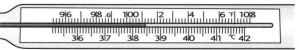

1. _____

2. _____

3. _____

4. _____

5. _____

5. Explain pulse and respirations

Matching
Use each letter only once.

1. _____ Apnea

2. ____ BPM

3. ____ Bradycardia

4. ____ Cheyne-Stokes respiration

5. ____ Dilate

6. ____ Dyspnea

7. ____ Eupnea

8. ____ Expiration

9. ____ Inspiration

10. ____ Orthopnea

11. ____ Respiration

12. ____ Tachycardia

13. ____ Tachypnea

(A) The absence of breathing

(B) To widen

(C) The process of inhaling air into the lungs and exhaling air out of the lungs

(D) Difficulty breathing

(E) The process of inhaling air into the lungs

(F) Slow heart rate—under 60 beats per minute

(G) Medical abbreviation for beats per minute

(H) The process of exhaling air out of the lungs

(I) Shortness of breath when lying down that is relieved by sitting up

(J) Type of respiration with periods of apnea lasting at least 10 seconds, along with alternating periods of slow, irregular respirations and rapid, shallow respirations

(K) Fast heartbeat—over 100 beats per minute

(L) Normal respirations

(M) Rapid respirations—over 20 breaths per minute

6. List guidelines for taking pulse and respirations

Multiple Choice

1. The most common site for counting pulse beats is:
   (A) Apical pulse
   (B) Radial pulse
   (C) Brachial pulse
   (D) Femoral pulse

2. Respiration rate is counted directly after taking the pulse because:
   (A) People tend to breathe more quickly if they know they are being observed.
   (B) People tend to breathe more slowly if they know they are being observed.
   (C) Breathing tends to be more regular if the person knows they are being observed.
   (D) It saves time for the nursing assistant.

3. If the radial pulse is less than the apical pulse, this may indicate:
   (A) Heart disease
   (B) Infection
   (C) Fever
   (D) Poor circulation to extremities

7. Identify factors that affect blood pressure

Crossword Puzzle

Across

3. Regular amounts of this usually decreases a person's blood pressure

5. Medical term for high blood pressure (140/90 or higher)

6. Top number in a blood pressure reading

7. Medical term for blood pressure that is 100/60 or lower

Down

1. Sudden drop in blood pressure when a person stands up

2. Bottom number in a blood pressure reading

4. Not having hypertension now but being likely to have it in the future

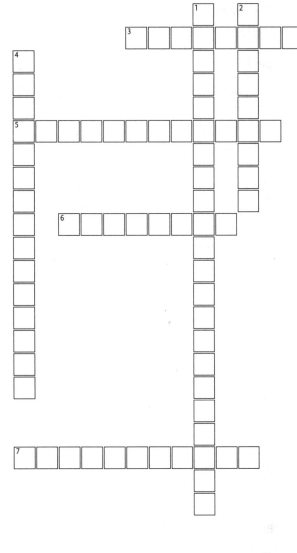

8. List guidelines for taking blood pressure

True or False

1. _____ Blood pressure is measured with a device called a sphygmomanometer.

2. _____ As long as a stethoscope is used, the placement of the cuff on the arm does not matter.

3. _____ An aneroid sphygmomanometer displays readings digitally.

4. _____ The apical pulse is the most commonly used pulse site to take a blood pressure reading.

5. _____ A blood pressure reading should not be taken on an arm that has a cast or is being used for dialysis.

6. _____ Blood pressure readings may be taken while a resident is lying down, sitting, and standing if he has orthostatic hypotension.

9. Describe guidelines for pain management

Short Answer

1. Have you ever been in pain for an extended period of time? If so, how did it affect your life?

_____

_____

_____

_____

_____

_____

_____

_____

2. Why is pain called the "fifth vital sign?"

_____

_____

_____

_____

3. List five questions that a nursing assistant should ask when helping a resident manage pain.

_____

_____

_____

_____

_____

_____

_____

_____

4. List ten signs that a resident is in pain.

_____

_____

_____

_____

_____

_____

_____

_____

_____

_____

Fill in the Blank

Looking at measures to reduce pain, fill in each of the following blanks.

1. Offer warm _____
   or _____.

2. Be _____,
   caring, gentle, and _____.

3. Offer _____
   frequently.

4. Assist in frequent changes of
   _____.

5. Report any complaints of _____
   or _____
   promptly to the nurse.

14

Nutrition and Fluid Balance

1. Review the key terms in Learning Objective 1 before completing the workbook exercises

2. Describe common nutritional problems of the elderly and the chronically ill

Crossword Puzzle

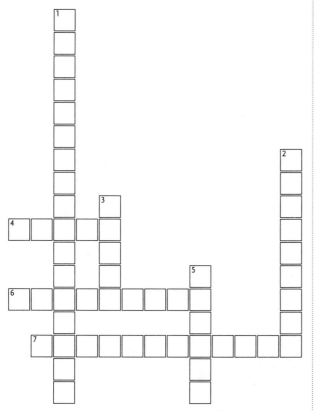

Across

4. One sense affected by aging and/or medication that affects the appetite

6. The medical term for difficulty swallowing

7. Lack of proper nutrition that results from insufficient food intake or an improper diet

Down

1. One disease that can make swallowing difficult

2. The taking in and using of food by the body to maintain health

3. Problems with these make chewing difficult

5. When less of this is produced, eating and swallowing are affected

3. Describe cultural factors that influence food preferences

Short Answer

1. List three factors that influence food choices.

_____

_____

_____

_____

_____

_____

_____

_____

_____

_____

_____

Name: _____

2. Of the factors you listed above, which one has the most influence on your personal food choices?

_____

_____

_____

_____

_____

_____

_____

_____

_____

4. Identify six basic nutrients

Short Answer

Write the letter of the correct basic nutrient beside each description below. Use a "W" for water, "F" for fats, "C" for carbohydrates, "P" for proteins, "V" for vitamins, or "M" for minerals. Letters may be used more than once.

1. _____ Essential for tissue growth and repair

2. _____ A person can survive only a few days without this

3. _____ Monounsaturated and polyunsaturated are types of this

4. _____ The body does not make most of these nutrients; they can only be obtained through certain foods

5. _____ Give flavor to foods

6. _____ Add fiber to diets, which helps with solid waste elimination

7. _____ Help keep bones and teeth strong

8. _____ Help remove waste products from cells

9. _____ Some of these are fat-soluble; some are water-soluble

10. _____ Most essential nutrient for life

5. Explain the USDA's MyPlate

Short Answer

The USDA developed the MyPlate icon and web address to help promote healthy eating practices. Looking at the MyPlate icon, fill in the food groups.

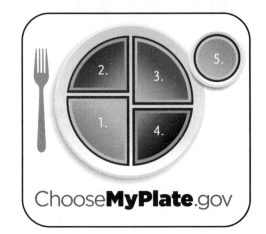

ChooseMyPlate.gov

1. _____

2. _____

3. _____

4. _____

5. _____

Short Answer

Read the following descriptions and mark which each is describing – "V" for vegetables, "F" for fruits, "G" for grains, "P" for protein, and "D" for dairy. Letters will be used more than once.

1. _____ This group includes foods that retain their calcium content, such as yogurt and cheese.

2. _____ This includes all foods made from wheat, rice, oats, cornmeal, and barley.

3. _____ Plant sources of this include beans and soy products.

4. _____ Eating seafood twice a week in place of meat or poultry is recommended for this group.

5. _____ Most choices from this group should be fat-free or low-fat.

6. _____ Important sources of dietary fiber and many nutrients, including folic acid and vitamin C.

7. ____ Half of a person's plate should consist of choices from these two groups.

8. ____ At least half of all of these consumed should be "whole."

9. ____ One subgroup of these contains the bran, germ, and endosperm.

10. ____ These products contain calcium, potassium, vitamin D, and protein.

11. ____ Within this group, dark green, red, and orange types have the best nutritional content.

12. ____ Animal sources of this include meat, poultry, seafood, and eggs.

Short Answer

1. What is calorie balance?

_____

_____

_____

_____

_____

2. What are two things that can help a person eat less?

_____

_____

_____

_____

3. List four types of foods that a person should eat more often.

_____

_____

_____

_____

4. List three types of food to eat less often.

_____

_____

_____

_____

5. List six types of food that are high in sodium.

_____

_____

_____

_____

_____

_____

_____

_____

_____

_____

6. What should be consumed instead of sugary drinks?

_____

_____

_____

6. Explain the role of the dietary department

Multiple Choice

1. Which of the following is a responsibility of the dietary department?
   (A) The department writes the medical order for which type of special diet each resident requires.
   (B) The department prepares food in such a way that residents are able to manage.
   (C) The department is responsible for making sure that residents are ready for their meals.
   (D) The department prepares food for residents' families.

2. Which of the following information is included on a resident's diet card?
   (A) Special diets, allergies, likes and dislikes, and other dietary instructions
   (B) Intake and output records
   (C) Amount of activity
   (D) Health department survey results

3. Which of the following is a guideline for reading menus to residents and assisting them with selecting their choices?
   (A) Speak quickly and loudly.
   (B) Do not include beverage choices.
   (C) Make selections sound appetizing.
   (D) Encourage nutritious choices, but make the final decision, even if resident prefers something else.

7. Explain the importance of following diet orders and identify special diets

Short Answer
For each of the following, list the kind of special diet it is describing.

1. Resident is drinking fluids that you can see through.

   _____

2. Resident has kidney or liver disease and is eating vegetables and starches and reducing protein intake.

   _____

3. Resident is eating whole grains and raw fruits and vegetables.

   _____

4. Resident is trying to lose or maintain weight.

   _____

5. Resident is making the transition from a liquid diet to a regular diet.

   _____

6. Resident has severe heart or kidney disease and has fluid intake monitored.

   _____

7. Resident has a serious burn that is healing and is eating meat, fish, and cheese.

   _____

8. Resident is taking diuretics and eating bananas, oranges, and sweet potatoes and yams.

   _____

9. Resident has trouble chewing and swallowing and cannot tolerate a regular or soft mechanical diet.

   _____

10. Resident has heart disease and is limiting his salt intake.

    _____

11. Resident has a bowel disorder and is decreasing intake of grains, dairy, and coffee.

    _____

12. Resident is consuming clear liquids with the addition of cream soups, milk, and ice cream.

    _____

13. Resident's food is prepared with a blender or food processor.

    _____

14. Resident has intestinal problems and is avoiding spicy foods and citrus fruits.

    _____

15. Resident is trying to gain weight after surgery or an illness.

    _____

16. Resident has heart disease and is eating white meat, skim milk, and low-fat cottage cheese.

    _____

17. Resident has a meal plan that must be followed exactly and must eat everything that is served.

    _____

18. Resident has celiac disease and foods containing wheat flour are eliminated from the diet.

_____

19. Resident cannot digest the sugar found in milk and other products, but is allowed soy milk.

_____

20. Resident does not eat meat for ethical reasons, but chooses to eat eggs and dairy products.

_____

21. Resident does not eat meat, poultry, fish, eggs, or dairy products.

_____

8. Explain thickened liquids and identify three basic thickening consistencies

True or False

1. _____ Residents with dysphagia are evaluated to determine if they should consume thickened liquids.

2. _____ Thickened liquids move down the throat more slowly and limit the risk of choking.

3. _____ Residents who need to consume thickened liquids are still allowed to drink non-thickened coffee and water.

4. _____ The three types of thickened liquids generally used by facilities are nectar thick, honey thick, and pudding thick.

5. _____ Residents can drink liquids that are pudding thick from a cup with or without a straw.

9. List ways to identify and prevent unintended weight loss

Fill in the Blank

1. Unintended weight loss may be due to a(n) _____ condition or a(n) _____ diet.

2. Unintended weight loss puts a person at a greater risk for _____.

3. It is important to _____ any weight loss you notice.

4. Staff may re-evaluate special _____ orders.

5. Warning signs of unintended weight loss include resident having _____ that do not fit properly or difficulty chewing or _____.

6. Signs that a resident is malnourished include a feeling of _____ throughout the body, weight loss, frequent _____ and problems with _____.

7. Report any decrease in _____ to the nurse.

8. _____ food to the resident's preferences.

9. Check _____ and trays to make sure residents are receiving the correct food.

10. Talk about food being served in a _____ way to encourage eating.

10. Describe how to make dining enjoyable for residents

True or False

1. _____ Mealtimes are often the most anticipated times of the day for residents.

2. _____ Nursing assistants should encourage residents to eat as little as possible so that they do not gain too much weight.

3. _____ Meals do not need to be served at the same time every day.

4. _____ Staff should honor residents' requests to sit with friends.

5. _____ The best position for eating is reclining 45 degrees.

Name: _____

6. ____ Dining tables should be adjusted to the right height for wheelchairs.

7. ____ Food should be served promptly to maintain correct temperature.

8. ____ Residents should be given assistive devices for eating, if needed.

9. ____ If a resident needs his food cut for him before eating, this should be done at the dining table.

10. ____ Residents must eat whatever food is served, even if it is not what they want.

11. Describe how to serve meal trays and assist with eating

Multiple Choice

1. When serving meals to residents, a nursing assistant should:
   (A) Check the diet card and identify the resident before serving the meal tray
   (B) Do as much as possible for each resident so that the meal can be finished more quickly
   (C) Leave the door of the food cart open so that the food is not too hot when served
   (D) Serve one resident at each table before going back to serve the second resident at each table

2. Which of the following is a way that a nursing assistant can promote residents' dignity during mealtime?
   (A) The nursing assistant should let residents know which food they need to eat first.
   (B) The nursing assistant should insist that residents wear bibs to keep their clothing free of food.
   (C) The nursing assistant should discourage conversation during mealtimes so that residents will be able to eat more quickly.
   (D) The nursing assistant should say positive things about the food being served.

3. Which of the following is a guideline that a nursing assistant should follow for helping residents during mealtime?
   (A) The nursing assistant should mix all of the food on the plate together so that residents will be more likely to eat it.
   (B) The nursing assistant should tell residents which foods look appetizing and which do not.
   (C) The nursing assistant should blow on food that is too hot to get it to cool down more quickly.
   (D) The nursing assistant should respect residents' refusals to eat but report them to the nurse.

4. In which position should a resident be for eating?
   (A) Partially reclining
   (B) Sitting upright
   (C) Flat on his or her back
   (D) On his or her side with the head raised

12. Describe how to assist residents with special needs

Short Answer
For each of the following problems with eating, list one technique for helping a resident to eat.

1. Resident has had a stroke and has a weaker side.

   _____

   _____

   _____

2. Resident has Parkinson's disease.

   _____

   _____

   _____

3. Resident is visually impaired.

   _____

   _____

   _____

4. Resident eats too quickly.

   _____

_____

_____

5.   Resident bites down on utensils.

_____

_____

6.   Resident cannot or will not chew.

_____

_____

7.   Resident will not stop chewing.

_____

_____

8.   Resident holds food in his mouth or will not swallow.

_____

_____

9.   Resident pockets food in his cheek.

_____

_____

10. Resident has poor lip closure.

_____

_____

11. Resident has no teeth or is missing teeth.

_____

_____

12. Resident has dentures that do not fit properly.

_____

_____

13. Resident has a change in vision.

_____

_____

14. Resident has a protruding tongue or tongue thrust.

_____

_____

15. Resident will not open mouth.

_____

_____

16. Resident falls asleep while eating.

_____

_____

17. Resident chokes when drinking.

_____

_____

18. Resident forgets to eat.

_____

_____

19. Resident drools excessively.

_____

_____

20. Resident has poor sitting balance.

_____

_____

21. Resident tends to lean to one side.

_____

_____

22. Resident tends to fall forward.

_____

_____

_____

23. Resident has poor neck control.

_____

_____

_____

13. Discuss dysphagia and list guidelines for preventing aspiration

Multiple Choice

1. Which of the following is a cause of dysphagia?
   (A) Problems with dentures
   (B) Problems with casts
   (C) Problems with splints
   (D) Problems with warm applications

2. Which of the following is a sign of dysphagia?
   (A) Eating very rapidly
   (B) Healthy enjoyment of eating
   (C) Normal breathing
   (D) Coughing during or after meals

3. Guidelines for preventing aspiration include:
   (A) Put residents in a reclining position for eating and drinking.
   (B) Place food in the paralyzed side of the mouth.
   (C) Offer at least three bites of food before offering a liquid.
   (D) Make sure food is swallowed after each bite.

14. Describe intake and output (I&O)

Short Answer

1. A healthy person generally needs to take in about 64 ounces (oz.) of fluid each day. How many milliliters (mL) is this?

_____

2. Ms. Brown just ate some butterscotch pudding from a 6-ounce container. You measure the leftover pudding, which is about 35 milliliters. How many milliliters (mL) of pudding did Ms. Brown eat?

_____

3. Record this resident's total intake and output:

   1 glass apple juice   140 mL
   1 cup coffee   110 mL
   1 cup soup   170 mL
   Total intake: _____

   11:00 a.m.
   Urinate x 1   220 mL output measured
   1:00 pm
   Urinate x 1   260 mL output measured
   Total output: _____

15. List ways to identify and prevent dehydration

Short Answer

1. What is dehydration?

_____

_____

_____

_____

2. List ten signs and symptoms of dehydration.

_____

_____

_____

_____

_____

_____

_____

_____

_____

_____

_____

_____

_____

3. Fill in the POURR acronym for encouraging fluids:

P _____

O _____

U _____

R _____

R _____

4. What should a nursing assistant do every time she sees a resident to help prevent dehydration?

_____

_____

_____

5. How could the water pitcher and cup being too heavy for a resident to lift contribute to dehydration?

_____

_____

_____

_____

_____

16. List signs and symptoms of fluid overload and describe conditions that may require fluid restrictions

Word Search

1. Fluid overload occurs when more fluid _____ the body than is _____ from the body.

2. Fluid overload can occur when the heart, _____, or lungs are not working properly.

3. Symptoms of fluid overload include weight _____, difficulty _____, and _____ heart rate.

4. Check for _____of the ankles, feet, fingers or hands.

5. _____ is swelling of the abdomen due to excess fluid.

6. Treating fluid overload consists of reduction in _____, increasing the number of _____ used for sleep, and _____ to eliminate the excessive fluid.

7. A(n) _____ order means the person must limit the daily amount of fluids to a level set by the doctor.

8. Reasons for fluid restrictions include recent _____, a special _____ ordered, or _____ through a special tube.

r	u	n	t	c	w	e	x	m	k	x	a	n	k
s	e	k	s	b	t	a	q	c	t	b	x	o	y
f	b	s	e	t	i	c	s	a	d	m	e	g	k
e	b	r	t	d	h	t	c	z	e	m	b	a	s
e	q	e	l	r	x	t	b	d	k	r	c	i	j
d	e	t	a	n	i	m	i	l	e	g	s	n	l
i	r	n	c	v	v	c	a	a	p	x	s	c	f
n	o	e	i	x	i	t	t	y	i	y	y	r	c
g	i	t	d	n	b	h	g	f	l	l	e	e	o
t	y	k	e	q	i	o	j	x	l	f	n	a	q
w	n	k	m	n	h	o	t	w	o	u	d	s	n
s	u	r	g	e	r	y	f	z	w	y	i	e	l
f	v	g	n	i	l	l	e	w	s	r	k	d	c
u	f	h	d	l	m	g	e	v	z	r	g	z	s

15

The Gastrointestinal System

1. Review the key terms in Learning Objective 1 before completing the workbook exercises

2. Explain key terms related to the body

Matching
Use each letter only once.

1. _____ Anatomy

2. _____ Biology

3. _____ Body systems

4. _____ Cells

5. _____ Homeostasis

6. _____ Organs

7. _____ Pathophysiology

8. _____ Physiology

9. _____ Tissues

(A) Groups of cells that perform specific body functions; connective and nervous are examples

(B) The study of all life forms

(C) Structural units in the body that perform specific functions; the heart is an example

(D) The study of body structure

(E) The study of the disorders that occur in the body

(F) The condition in which all of the body's systems are balanced and working at their best

(G) Basic structural unit of all organisms

(H) Groups of organs that perform specific functions in the body

(I) The study of how body parts function

3. Explain the structure and function of the gastrointestinal system

Word Search

1. The gastrointestinal system is made up of two sections: the

   _____

   and the _____

   _____.

2. Most food and fluids are absorbed in the

   _____.

3. The epiglottis blocks food from entering the

   _____.

4. Feces is eliminated from the body by

   _____ through

   the anus.

5. The large intestine helps regulate water balance by absorbing _____

   and _____ and

   eliminating solid waste as feces.

6. The functions of the gastrointestinal system are _____ and

   _____ of food,

   absorption of nutrients, and

   _____ of waste

   products.

Name: _____

```
e o a t p b a k g r u t o w
z u c c m d l d u j i u c d
c s c a i z b b s l i o q r
t p e r i s t a l s i s g y
y u s t t o u b l h q w m i
g a s l y f m v h t j f k r
u i o a a l i u t w i n y j
e n r n i x o r q u o q u z
i n y i v a a r a i j q o q
a s o t t c e j t y j p r m
o r r s h t s s x c b p j m
u f g e k v e r d m e e c m
f g a t t g l c x z c l t e
k j n n a s i e m h i e a
z s s i o t w l s v w m z u
r d w o i c c e g t a i c l
h z o r t m j p q u c n o h
e n i t s e t n i l l a m s
h j u s e y q s t f t t b d
b m g a g t c u z r g i y d
p j y g i e o o l u s o i q
x o h o d y h x r d l n o n
```

4. Discuss changes in the gastrointestinal system due to aging

True or False

1. _____ As a person ages, he may find it harder to taste foods.

2. _____ An older person may be constipated more often.

3. _____ Difficulty chewing and swallowing may occur as a person ages.

4. _____ An increase in the ability to absorb vitamins and minerals is a normal change of aging.

5. _____ As a person ages, she may have an increase of saliva and other digestive fluids.

5. List normal qualities of stool and identify signs and symptoms to report about stool

Multiple Choice

1. Solid waste products eliminated by the colon are called:
   (A) Tarry
   (B) Feces
   (C) Peristalsis
   (D) Chyme

2. What should normal stool look like?
   (A) It should be brown and formed.
   (B) It should be brown and loose.
   (C) It should be brown and hard.
   (D) It should be brown and liquid.

3. Which of the following is true of bowel elimination?
   (A) There should not be any pain with passing stool.
   (B) All people have a bowel movement once per day.
   (C) Fecal incontinence is a normal part of aging.
   (D) It is normal for blood to be in a person's stool.

6. List factors affecting bowel elimination and describe how to promote normal bowel elimination

Short Answer

1. List one way each of these factors affects bowel elimination: growth and development, psychological factors, diet, fluid intake, physical activity and exercise, personal habits, and medications.

_____

_____

_____

_____

_____

_____

_____

_____
_____
_____
_____
_____
_____
_____
_____
_____
_____
_____
_____
_____

2. What is the difference between a standard bedpan and a fracture pan? How should each be placed?

_____
_____
_____
_____
_____
_____

7. Discuss common disorders of the gastrointestinal system

Matching
For each of the following descriptions, write the letter of the disorder to which it refers. Use each letter only once.

1. _____ Causes the wall of the intestines (large or small) to become inflamed

2. _____ Frequent elimination of liquid or semi-liquid feces

3. _____ Results from a weakening of the sphincter muscle which joins the esophagus and the stomach; also known as acid reflux

4. _____ Enlarged veins in the rectum that can cause itching, burning, pain and bleeding

5. _____ Raw sores in the stomach and small intestine

6. _____ Sac-like pouchings of the intestinal wall develop in weakened areas of the wall of the large intestine

7. _____ Chronic condition of the gastrointestinal tract that is worsened by stress

8. _____ Chronic condition in which the liquid contents of the stomach back up into the esophagus

9. _____ Mass of dry, hard stool that remains packed in the rectum and cannot be expelled

10. _____ Nutrients from the intestinal tract are not properly absorbed

11. _____ Inability to control the muscles of the bowels, leading to involuntary passage of stool or gas

12. _____ Inflammation of and sores in the lining of the large intestine; is a form of inflammatory bowel disease (IBD)

13. _____ Inflammation of sacs that develop in the wall of the large intestine due to diverticulosis

14. _____ Inability to eliminate stool, or the infrequent, difficult, and often painful elimination of a hard, dry stool

15. _____ Air in the intestine that is passed through the rectum

(A) Constipation

(B) Crohn's disease

(C) Diarrhea

(D) Diverticulitis

(E) Diverticulosis

(F) Fecal impaction

(G) Fecal incontinence

(H) Flatulence

(I) Gastroesophageal reflux disease (GERD)

(J) Heartburn

(K) Hemorrhoids

(L) Irritable bowel syndrome

(M) Malabsorption

(N) Ulcerative colitis

(O) Ulcers

8. Discuss how enemas are given

Fill in the Blank

1. An enema is given when help is needed

    _____

    from the colon.

2. Enemas are also ordered in preparation for

    a(n) _____ or

    _____.

3. _____ water,

    _____ and

    _____ enemas

    are considered cleansing enemas.

4. _____

    enemas require more fluid than

    _____ enemas.

5. Remove the _____

    from tubing before inserting it into the rec-

    tum.

6. During the enema, the resident should be in

    the _____ position.

7. Stop immediately if the resident has

    _____ or if

    you feel resistance.

8. Observe for _____,

    pain or discomfort, bleeding, and the ability

    to _____ the fluid.

9. The goals of using an oil-retention enema

    include lubricating the intestine, soften-

    ing _____, and reducing

    _____ with bowel

    movements.

9. Demonstrate how to collect a stool specimen

True or False

1. ____ A specimen is a sample used for anal-
    ysis and diagnosis.

2. ____ A stool sample may be tested for
    blood, pathogens, or other things.

3. ____ If testing stool for ova and parasites,
    leave it in the refrigerator overnight
    before taking it to the lab.

4. ____ Specimens are stored in the same
    refrigerators that are used for food
    and drinks.

5. ____ Urine and toilet paper should not be
    included in a stool specimen.

6. ____ A plastic collection container called
    a "hat" is sometimes inserted into a
    toilet to collect and measure urine or
    stool.

7. ____ Collecting a specimen from a resident
    in isolation requires the same proce-
    dure as is used for a resident who is
    not in isolation.

10. Explain occult blood testing

Fill in the Blank

1. Hidden or _____
    blood is found inside stool with a

    _____ or

    a special _____
    test.

2. Blood in stool may be a sign of a serious
    physical problem such as

    _____.

3. The _____
    test checks for occult blood in stool.

4. Specific _____ orders or
    _____ may be

    necessary prior to testing.

11. Define the term "ostomy" and identify the difference between colostomy and ileostomy

Short Answer

1. List one reason why an ostomy might be necessary.

_____

_____

2. List three ways to help a person with an ostomy feel better about himself.

_____

_____

_____

_____

_____

_____

_____

_____

_____

12. Explain guidelines for assisting with bowel retraining

Crossword Puzzle

Across

3. The process of assisting residents to regain control of their bowels or bladder

5. Being this way is the opposite of being negative

6. Can be offered at specific times each day

7. Nursing assistants must answer these promptly during the retraining process

Down

1. Wearing gloves while handling body wastes is a part of these

2. Predict bathroom times by observing these

4. Providing this as needed helps promote proper hygiene

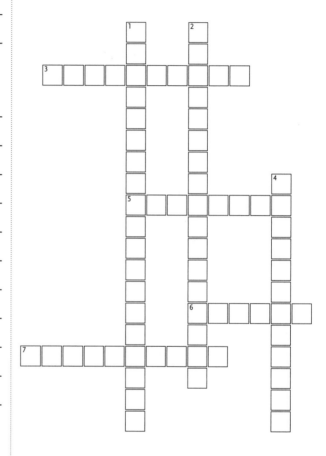

16

The Urinary System

1. Review the key terms in Learning Objective 1 before completing the workbook exercises

2. Explain the structure and function of the urinary system

Fill in the Blank

1. The kidneys clean and _____ waste products and _____ materials from the blood.

2. The urinary system consists of two _____, two _____, the urinary bladder, and the meatus.

3. Substances not needed by the body—toxins and waste products—stay in the kidneys and form _____.

4. The female urethra is _____ than the male urethra.

5. The functions of the urinary system are elimination of _____ products from the blood, maintenance of _____ in the body, regulation of the levels of electrolytes in the body, and assistance in regulation of blood pressure.

3. Discuss changes in the urinary system due to aging

True or False

1. _____ Kidneys not filtering blood as efficiently is a normal change of aging.

2. _____ As people age, the bladder holds more urine than it used to.

3. _____ Bladder muscle tone weakens with age.

4. _____ The bladder may not empty completely as a person ages, increasing the chance of infection.

4. List normal qualities of urine and identify signs and symptoms to report about urine

Multiple Choice

1. What should normal urine look like?
   (A) It should be cloudy.
   (B) It should be pale yellow.
   (C) It should be dark brown.
   (D) It should be light red.

2. How many milliliters (mL) of urine do adults normally produce?
   (A) 900 to 1000 mL
   (B) 500 to 1000 mL
   (C) 200 to 400 mL
   (D) 1200 to 1500 mL

3. Which of the following statements is true of urine and urination?
   (A) People urinate several times a day to remain healthy.
   (B) Urinary incontinence is a normal part of getting older.
   (C) People normally urinate twice a day to remain healthy.
   (D) Burning during urination is to be expected as a person ages.

5. List factors affecting urination and describe how to promote normal urination

Short Answer
List one way each of these factors affects urination: growth and development, psychological factors, fluid intake, physical activity and exercise, personal habits, medications, and disorders.

6. Discuss common disorders of the urinary system

Matching
For each of the following descriptions, write the letter of the disorder to which it refers. Use each letter only once.

1. ＿＿＿ Process that cleans the body of wastes that the kidneys cannot remove due to kidney failure

2. ＿＿＿ Inability to adequately or completely empty the bladder

3. ＿＿＿ Progressive condition in which the kidneys cannot filter certain waste products from the blood

4. ＿＿＿ Usually occurs when bacteria enter the urinary tract through the urethra and then begin to multiply in the bladder

5. ＿＿＿ Condition in which kidneys have failed and dialysis or transplantation is required to sustain life

(A) Chronic renal failure (CRF)

(B) Dialysis

(C) End-stage renal disease (ESRD)

(D) Urinary tract infection (UTI)

(E) Urine retention

7. Discuss reasons for incontinence

Crossword Puzzle

Across

4. An emotion that urinary incontinence can cause

5. It should be left within reach and answered promptly

6. Another name for incontinence pad

Down

1. To prevent skin breakdown, nursing assistants should give this type of care as often as needed

2. The inability to control the muscles of the bladder, which leads to an involuntary loss of urine

3. Not exposing residents and keeping voices low when discussing incontinence are part of providing for this legal right for residents

4. Something that nursing assistants should encourage plenty of

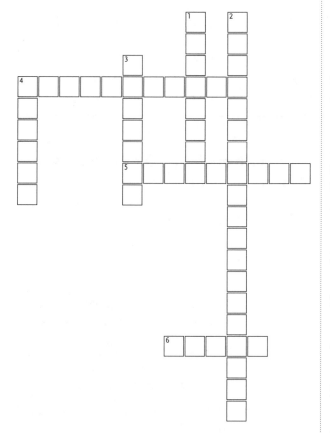

8. Describe catheters and related care

Multiple Choice

1. A catheter that stays in the bladder for a period of time is called:
   (A) Straight catheter
   (B) Indwelling catheter
   (C) Condom catheter
   (D) Texas catheter

2. What is the nursing assistant's role regarding catheters?
   (A) Giving daily catheter care
   (B) Inserting the catheter
   (C) Irrigating the catheter
   (D) Removing the catheter

3. Which of the following statements is true of providing catheter care?
   (A) The nursing assistant should give daily care of the genital area to keep it clean.
   (B) The nursing assistant should make sure the drainage bag hangs higher then the level of the hips or bladder.
   (C) The nursing assistant should store the drainage bag on the floor.
   (D) The nursing assistant should re-attach the catheter tube when it has disconnected.

9. Explain how to collect different types of urine specimens

Matching
For each of the following descriptions, write the letter of the specimen to which it refers. Some letters will be used more than once.

1. _____ Collects all urine voided by resident during a 24-hour period

2. _____ First and last urine voided is not included in the sample

3. _____ May be done when a resident has urinary retention

4. _____ Obtained when a resident cannot urinate on his or own

5. _____ Can be collected any time resident voids

6. _____ When beginning test, resident must void and discard first urine

(A) 24-hour urine specimen

(B) Catheterized urine specimen

(C) Clean-catch urine specimen

(D) Routine urine specimen

Short Answer

1. How is a specimen collected from a resident with a urostomy?

_____

_____

_____

Name: _____

_____

_____

_____

_____

2. List the five "rights" of specimen collection.

_____

_____

_____

_____

_____

_____

```
m j q r g z c y h m a b l k
g u k e t o n e s a e s i d
m c x a n r h l w k t j k z
r z p g h i c s p a w r g s
g s s e n l l i n a z d f c
f r y n d m x a j f z p a i
g a e t i y u d k s l r t s
u g n d i l u t e l p k u u
k u d s v v u c p n a k m h
l s i n j j a s o j s j x m
l t k w m z x r n q v e f r
d c l z g w d m g i q n z n
o m w r f q i w c u w n r t
e h l j u m c x u o x w b t
```

10. Explain types of tests that are performed on urine

Word Search

1. Dip strips, also called _____ strips, test urine for glucose, pH level, ketones, blood, and specific

   _____.

2. The higher the pH level of a fluid, the more _____ the fluid is.

3. Without _____ to process glucose, _____ build up in the blood and spill into the urine.

4. _____ and _____ can cause blood to appear in urine.

5. A specific gravity test is done to make sure the _____ are functioning properly.

6. Urine can be very _____, or close to water; it can also be very _____, or concentrated.

11. Explain guidelines for assisting with bladder retraining

True or False

1. _____ Loss of normal bladder function can be caused by illness, injury, or inactivity.

2. _____ Residents will not usually be embarrassed by episodes of incontinence.

3. _____ Observing residents' elimination habits helps predict when a trip to the bathroom may be necessary.

4. _____ Offer a trip to the bathroom, bedpan, or urinal before beginning procedures and after completing procedures.

5. _____ Residents who have problems with incontinence should be discouraged from drinking fluids.

6. _____ Telling a resident how frustrated you are when he is incontinent will encourage him to control his bladder.

7. _____ Residents must be encouraged to ask for help with elimination whenever they need it.

17

The Reproductive System

1. Review the key terms in Learning Objective 1 before completing the workbook exercises

2. Explain the structure and function of the reproductive system

Fill in the Blank

1. Ova are released from the ovaries each month during the process of
_____.

2. The male and female reproductive glands are called _____.

3. The female reproductive system produces the female sex cells and the female hormones, _____ and _____.

4. The female reproductive system is made up of the _____, fallopian tubes, uterus, _____,
the vulva, and the breasts.

5. The _____
receives sperm during intercourse and is the outlet for menstrual blood.

6. The male reproductive system consists of the _____, testes, scrotum, epididymis, vas deferens, _____ tissue, seminal vesicle, ejaculatory duct, and _____ gland.

7. If an ovum is fertilized, it moves into the
_____.

8. The male reproductive system produces the male hormone, _____.

9. Every milliliter of semen contains 50 to 150 million _____.

3. Discuss changes in the reproductive system due to aging

True or False

1. _____ A man's prostate gland enlarges with age.

2. _____ Menopause is a normal change of aging.

3. _____ A woman's production of estrogen and progesterone increases as she ages.

4. _____ Number and capability of sperm decrease with age.

5. _____ It takes less time for an older man to achieve an erection and to reach orgasm.

6. _____ As a woman ages, her vaginal walls become drier and thinner, which may cause discomfort during sexual intercourse.

4. Discuss common disorders of the reproductive system

Matching
For each of the following descriptions, write the letter of the disorder to which it refers. Use each letter only once.

1. _____ The prostate becomes enlarged and causes problems with urination

2. _____ Caused by bacteria and causes burning with urination, discharge from the penis or vagina, and low back pain

3. _____ Caused by a virus and cannot be cured; symptoms include itching and painful red blisters or open sores

Name: _____

4. ____ Inflammation of the vagina that causes vaginal discharge, itching and pain

5. ____ Green, cloudy, pus-like discharge from the penis and swelling of the testes; can cause sterility and pelvic inflammatory disease if not treated

6. ____ Caused by a virus, and genital warts may appear

7. ____ Caused by bacteria and small, painless sores on the penis may appear soon after infection

8. ____ Caused by protozoa and symptoms include a green-yellow vaginal discharge with a strong odor

(A) Benign prostatic hypertrophy (BPH)

(B) Chlamydia

(C) Genital herpes

(D) Genital HPV infection

(E) Gonorrhea

(F) Syphilis

(G) Trichomoniasis

(H) Vaginitis

5. Describe sexual needs of the elderly

Short Answer

1. What is the appropriate attitude for a nursing assistant to have regarding residents' sexual behaviors?

_____

_____

_____

_____

_____

_____

_____

2. What should a nursing assistant do if she encounters a sexual situation?

_____

_____

_____

6. Describe vaginal irrigation

Word Search

1. A vaginal _____ is a rinsing of the vagina to clean the vaginal tract.

2. It is performed prior to _____ procedures or examinations or due to vaginal _____.

3. Vaginal irrigations are also used to introduce _____ into the vagina to treat disorders or reduce _____ _____.

4. Always provide plenty of _____ for this procedure.

5. Place the resident in the _____ position.

6. Do not _____ the tip into the vagina.

7. Report pain or discomfort or _____ swelling to the nurse.

z	q	k	q	k	z	d	b	b	g	f	z	h	n
r	i	r	p	d	b	o	n	g	o	g	t	d	m
d	j	u	d	n	i	r	r	y	l	t	o	x	j
k	j	p	c	b	v	s	y	a	a	p	n	q	s
l	j	p	r	i	v	a	c	y	n	o	p	f	a
o	i	m	e	l	x	l	d	o	i	y	g	e	f
b	l	m	x	i	l	r	q	t	m	y	j	r	t
j	f	x	x	l	a	e	a	p	o	f	l	m	l
l	i	v	t	i	c	c	a	o	d	m	o	v	u
p	u	d	n	r	i	u	l	z	b	l	x	r	j
q	k	a	o	d	g	m	j	b	a	w	j	z	t
y	g	f	e	y	r	b	w	h	r	a	h	r	f
e	x	m	n	l	u	e	m	m	n	j	j	h	k
g	k	b	i	v	s	n	q	y	o	w	q	r	j
q	t	c	n	o	i	t	a	g	i	r	r	i	v

18

The Integumentary System

1. Review the key terms in Learning Objective 1 before completing the workbook exercises

2. Explain the structure and function of the integumentary system

Fill in the Blank

1. The skin is the largest _____ in the human body.

2. The substance that gives skin its color is

   _____.

3. The skin covers and _____ the body, provides _____ through nerves, regulates body temperature, and prevents the loss of too much

   _____.

4. The two basic layers of the skin are the
   _____ and
   the _____.

5. _____ are found in the skin that give us the ability to feel and touch.

Short Answer

1. List the parts of the integumentary system.

   _____

   _____

   _____

   _____

   _____

   _____

2. List five functions of the integumentary system.

   _____

   _____

   _____

   _____

   _____

   _____

   _____

   _____

   _____

   _____

3. Discuss changes in the integumentary system due to aging

True or False

1. ____ Skin cancer happens normally as a person ages.

2. ____ The amount of fat and collagen increases with age.

3. ____ Skin loses elasticity with age, causing wrinkles.

4. ____ Skin becoming thinner and more fragile is a normal change of aging.

5. ____ Nail growth slows as a person ages.

6. ____ Brown spots may appear on the skin in areas exposed to the sun.

7. ____ Hair becoming thicker is a normal change of aging.

4. Discuss common disorders of the integumentary system

Matching
For each of the following descriptions, write the letter of the disorder to which it refers. Use each letter only once.

1. _____ Caused by tiny mites that burrow into the skin to lay eggs

2. _____ Death of tissue caused by a lack of blood flow

3. _____ Rough, hard bumps caused by a virus that invades the skin, usually through a cut or tear

4. _____ Chronic skin condition in which cells of the skin grow too fast, causing red, white, or silver patches to form

5. _____ Commonly occurs in moist areas; yeast is one type

6. _____ Can be classified as superficial, partial-thickness, and full-thickness

7. _____ Caused by the same virus that causes chickenpox

8. _____ General term for variety of skin problems; also called dermatitis

9. _____ Fungal infection that causes red scaly patches to appear in a ring shape

10. _____ Growth of abnormal skin cells; most serious form is malignant melanoma

11. _____ Types of these include abrasions, avulsions, incisions, lacerations, punctures and contusions

(A) Burns

(B) Eczema

(C) Fungal infections

(D) Gangrene

(E) Psoriasis

(F) Scabies

(G) Shingles

(H) Skin cancer

(I) Tinea

(J) Warts

(K) Wounds

5. Discuss pressure ulcers and identify guidelines for preventing pressure ulcers

Word Search

1. Skin breakdown usually occurs at _____ points.

2. Areas of the body where the bone lies close to the skin are called _____ _____.

3. _____ is the death of living cells or tissues.

4. Moisture and _____ contribute to skin breakdown.

5. The sores or wounds that result from skin deterioration and shearing are called _____ _____.

6. The first signs of skin breakdown include pale, white, or _____ skin.

7. Pressure ulcers are much easier to _____ than to cure.

8. Darker skin may look _____ when skin breakdown begins to occur.

9. _____ linens, as well as crumbs or other irritating objects in the bed increase the risk of pressure ulcers.

10. Keep skin clean and _____.

11. Assist immobile residents to change position at least every _____ hours.

12. Perform _____ _____ exercises as ordered.

13. Use _____ to separate skin surfaces.

```
i  b  z  i  u  d  e  l  k  n  i  r  w  u
j  o  d  u  n  d  x  v  y  e  v  l  v  k
e  n  f  r  c  x  x  o  v  c  t  r  s  j
n  y  e  x  y  z  m  g  x  r  k  a  k  o
g  p  i  m  t  z  o  r  n  o  j  v  b  f
s  r  e  c  l  u  e  r  u  s  s  e  r  p
y  o  p  j  t  d  v  h  c  i  w  d  s  i
i  m  q  r  d  n  t  v  k  s  o  u  h  d
v  i  a  e  e  m  e  q  g  j  l  x  j  c
a  n  n  i  r  s  f  v  k  s  l  t  z  j
x  e  r  a  u  l  s  q  e  x  i  w  c  l
d  n  w  p  b  s  q  u  j  r  p  o  i  o
k  c  p  u  r  p  l  e  r  m  p  u  y  a
k  e  x  e  a  p  e  c  e  e  s  k  b  q
h  s  r  f  k  q  d  w  u  s  m  g  l  q
r  a  n  g  e  o  f  m  o  t  i  o  n  h
```

Short Answer

Briefly describe what happens in each of the four stages of pressure ulcers.

_____

_____

_____

_____

_____

_____

_____

_____

_____

_____

_____

_____

_____

_____

_____

_____

_____

_____

_____

_____

_____

_____

_____

_____

_____

_____

_____

_____

_____

_____

6. Explain the benefits of warm and cold applications

True or False

1. ____ Hot or cold applications can be either moist or dry.

2. ____ The body responds to both heat and cold in the same way.

3. ____ Warm applications close blood vessels, and cold applications open them.

4. ____ You should always wear gloves when assisting with a sitz bath.

5. ____ Moist applications are less likely to cause injury than dry applications.

6. ____ Residents with high temperatures may need to have a cooling or tepid sponge bath.

7. ____ Warm and cold applications should not be applied for more than 20 minutes at a time.

Name: _____

Multiple Choice

1. Benefits of using warm applications include:
   - (A) Heat relieves pain and decreases swelling.
   - (B) Heat decreases blood flow to the area.
   - (C) Heat helps stop bleeding.
   - (D) Heat constricts/closes blood vessels.

2. The benefits of using cold applications include:
   - (A) Cold dilates/opens blood vessels.
   - (B) Cold increases blood flow to the area.
   - (C) Cold brings down high temperatures.
   - (D) Cold makes skin cyanotic.

3. How does moisture affect warm and cold applications?
   - (A) Moisture strengthens the effect of heat and cold.
   - (B) Moisture weakens the effect of heat and cold.
   - (C) Moisture has no effect, just like dry applications.
   - (D) Moisture allows use of warm and cold applications for longer than 20 minutes.

4. Which of the following is true of sitz baths?
   - (A) Sitz baths are often ordered for people who have asthma.
   - (B) Sitz baths are given with the resident standing up.
   - (C) Sitz baths can cause the resident to feel weak and dizzy.
   - (D) Sitz baths are used for swelling of the feet and hands.

7. Discuss non-sterile and sterile dressings

Short Answer

1. How do open wounds increase the risk of infection?

   _____

   _____

   _____

   _____

   _____

2. When are non-sterile dressings applied to wounds? When are sterile dressings applied to wounds?

   _____

   _____

   _____

   _____

   _____

   _____

   _____

   _____

3. List three types of supplies that are considered sterile.

   _____

   _____

   _____

   _____

   _____

   _____

   _____

4. What happens if any part of a sterile field becomes contaminated?

   _____

   _____

   _____

   _____

   _____

   _____

   _____

19

The Circulatory or Cardiovascular System

1. Review the key terms in Learning Objective 1 before completing the workbook exercises

2. Explain the structure and function of the circulatory system

Word Search

1. The heart is composed of _____ main chambers: the _____ and the _____.

2. Carbon dioxide is removed in the _____ when we exhale, and _____ is added when we inhale.

3. Blood is made up of solids and liquids: _____ and _____.

4. Blood is pumped from the right _____ to the right ventricle.

5. Platelets cause the blood to _____, preventing excess _____.

6. The function of the heart is to _____ through the blood vessels to every cell.

7. A function of blood is to transport oxygen, _____, hormones, salts, and antibodies to cells.

8. Plasma is made up of mostly _____.

9. The largest artery in the body is the _____.

10. Blood is composed of three different types of blood cells: red blood cells or _____, white blood cells or _____, and platelets or _____.

11. _____ gives blood its red color.

c	c	f	l	j	f	m	f	s	k	l	w	z	g
y	a	t	r	o	a	w	s	k	d	m	t	n	a
k	j	a	s	b	x	j	i	e	w	u	i	b	g
a	i	k	n	r	j	y	q	c	f	d	g	i	x
s	c	u	a	f	x	j	g	t	e	o	r	d	h
c	e	a	f	v	v	p	r	e	h	o	p	d	f
h	l	t	r	q	r	j	l	m	n	l	o	h	v
m	l	r	y	n	x	b	m	a	n	b	b	d	e
v	s	i	d	c	o	s	b	v	s	p	k	l	n
h	f	a	w	t	o	l	c	s	d	m	e	i	t
w	a	n	x	z	v	b	u	e	k	u	a	p	r
i	m	h	a	d	n	f	m	n	k	p	w	d	i
k	r	u	o	f	m	s	z	o	g	c	x	f	c
m	u	f	i	g	u	s	c	m	r	s	e	o	l
q	e	a	k	r	w	y	e	r	d	h	w	g	e
b	w	e	r	y	t	h	r	o	c	y	t	e	s
z	k	k	r	e	t	a	w	h	q	k	d	j	l
g	a	m	s	d	s	t	n	e	i	r	t	u	n

3. Discuss changes in the circulatory system due to aging

True or False

1. _____ Heart disease is a normal part of aging.

2. ____ The heart pumping less efficiently is a normal part of aging.

3. ____ Blood vessels widen and become more efficient with age.

4. ____ Blood vessels become less elastic as a person ages.

5. ____ As a person gets older, blood flow increases.

4. Discuss common disorders of the circulatory system

Matching
For each of the following descriptions, write the letter of the disorder to which it refers. Use each letter only once.

1. ____ Occurs when the coronary arteries narrow, causing reduced blood supply to the heart

2. ____ Condition in which the amount of red blood cells or hemoglobin in the body is less than normal

3. ____ Help prevent swelling and blood clots and increase blood circulation

4. ____ Obstruction of a blood vessel

5. ____ All or part of the blood flow to the heart muscle is blocked, causing muscle cells to die

6. ____ Most common type of peripheral vascular disease (PVD)

7. ____ Chest pain, pressure, or discomfort due to CAD

8. ____ Lack of blood supply to an area

9. ____ Condition in which blood supply to the legs, feet, arms, or hands is decreased due to poor circulation

10. ____ Shortness of breath when lying down that is relieved by sitting up

11. ____ Occurs when normal cardiac output cannot meet the body's needs for activities of daily living (ADLs)

12. ____ Chest pain that occurs when person is active or under severe stress

13. ____ Chest pain that occurs when a person is at rest and not exerting himself

14. ____ Person does not have high blood pressure now but is likely to in the future

15. ____ Blood pressure consistently measuring 140/90 or higher

(A) Anemia

(B) Angina pectoris

(C) Anti-embolic stockings

(D) Congestive heart failure (CHF)

(E) Coronary artery disease (CAD)

(F) Hypertension (HTN)

(G) Ischemia

(H) Myocardial infarction (heart attack)

(I) Occlusion

(J) Orthopnea

(K) Peripheral arterial disease (PAD)

(L) Peripheral vascular disease (PVD)

(M) Prehypertension

(N) Stable angina

(O) Unstable angina

20

The Respiratory System

1. Review the key terms in Learning Objective 1 before completing the workbook exercises

2. Explain the structure and function of the respiratory system

Fill in the Blank

1. Two functions of the respiratory system are to _____ oxygen to cells and _____ carbon dioxide from the cells.

2. _____ is the process that consists of inspiration (breathing in) and expiration (breathing out).

3. The epiglottis blocks food from entering the windpipe, or _____.

4. The _____ contract and expand the chest cavity during _____, when we breathe in.

5. The larynx enables humans to _____.

6. The lungs are covered by a membrane called the _____.

7. The exchange of _____ and _____ gases occurs in the lungs and in the cells.

8. The process of breathing air in and out is _____; it never stops.

9. The air sacs of the lungs are called the _____.

Short Answer

1. List the parts of the respiratory system.

_____

_____

_____

_____

_____

_____

_____

_____

_____

2. List the four functions of the respiratory system.

_____

_____

_____

_____

_____

_____

_____

3. Discuss changes in the respiratory system due to aging

True or False

1. _____ A decrease in lung capacity is a normal change of aging.

2. ____ Asthma is a normal part of aging.

3. ____ As a person ages, the air sacs in the lungs become less elastic and decrease in number.

4. ____ Airways become more elastic with age, increasing movement of air inside the lungs.

5. ____ When a person gets older, his rib cage changes and the chest muscles become weaker.

6. ____ With age, the cough reflex becomes more effective, and coughs become stronger.

7. ____ Oxygen in blood decreases with age.

8. ____ A person's voice becomes weaker as she gets older.

4. Discuss common disorders of the respiratory system

Matching
For each of the following descriptions, write the letter of the disorder to which it refers. Use each letter only once.

1. ____ Type of bronchitis caused by an infection; usually treated with antibiotics

2. ____ Highly contagious lung disease that can cause death if left untreated

3. ____ Chronic, progressive disease leading to difficulty breathing due to obstruction of the airways

4. ____ Chronic, episodic disorder with unknown cause; residents may need an inhaler with them at all times

5. ____ Chronic condition that usually results from cigarette smoking and chronic bronchitis

6. ____ Can develop when a person with TB fails to take all of the prescribed medication

7. ____ Permanent dilation/widening of the bronchi that causes chronic coughing, shortness of breath, weight loss and coughing up blood

8. ____ Type of bronchitis in which the lining of bronchial tubes becomes inflamed, causing scarring of the lining of the bronchial tubes

9. ____ Inflammation of the lungs caused by viral, bacterial, or fungal infection and/or chemical irritants

(A) Acute bronchitis

(B) Asthma

(C) Bronchiectasis

(D) Chronic bronchitis

(E) Chronic obstructive pulmonary disease (COPD)

(F) Emphysema

(G) Multidrug-resistant TB (MDR-TB)

(H) Pneumonia

(I) Tuberculosis (TB)

5. Describe oxygen delivery

True or False

1. ____ Nursing assistants may remove a resident's oxygen if the resident requests it.

2. ____ It is safe to smoke around oxygen, as long as it is not done within two feet of the oxygen device.

3. ____ Oxygen therapy is the administration of oxygen given to increase the supply of oxygen to the lungs.

4. ____ Oxygen can be adjusted by nursing assistants when the oxygen equipment does not seem to be working.

5. ____ Common types of oxygen delivery devices include the nasal cannula, simple face mask, and the oxygen concentrator.

6. ____ It is important to perform frequent skin care on areas of the face on which an oxygen device rests.

7. ____ Petroleum-based lubricants are best for soothing sensitive areas on the nose and mouth when a person is using oxygen.

8. ____ A nursing assistant should encourage activity as permitted for residents who are receiving oxygen.

9. ____ Notify the nurse of sores on the nasal area, complaints of discomfort or pain, and chest pain or tightness.

10. ____ All residents using oxygen will need oxygen continuously.

6. Describe how to collect a sputum specimen

Crossword Puzzle

Across

5. Best time of the day to collect sputum

6. Comes from the salivary glands and is not the same as sputum

Down

1. One of the things that a sputum specimen is checked for

2. Mucus that comes from inside the respiratory system

3. Use this to rinse the mouth before obtaining a sputum specimen

4. Fluid that should not be used for rinsing the mouth before a sputum collection

7. Describe the benefits of deep breathing exercises

Short Answer

1. Why might residents need to do deep breathing exercises?

_____

_____

_____

_____

_____

_____

2. List two possible benefits of regular use of the incentive spirometer.

_____

_____

_____

_____

_____

_____

_____

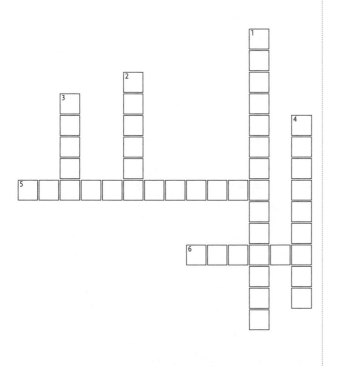

21

The Musculoskeletal System

1. Review the key terms in Learning Objective 1 before completing the workbook exercises

2. Explain the structure and function of the musculoskeletal system

Fill in the Blank

1. The musculoskeletal system gives the body _____ and _____.

2. The musculoskeletal system allows the body to _____ and _____ itself, provides _____ for the body and creates _____.

3. Muscles are groups of _____ that help the body move by _____ and _____.

4. _____ are the rigid connective tissues that make up the _____, which is the framework of the human body.

5. _____ are found at the place where two bones come together; they hold bones together and provide movement and _____.

6. _____ are strong, fibrous bands that connect bones and help _____ the joints and joint movement.

Short Answer

1. List the five parts of the musculoskeletal system.

_____

_____

_____

_____

_____

_____

_____

2. List the three types of muscles in the body.

_____

_____

_____

_____

_____

_____

_____

_____

3. List the four types of bones.

_____

_____

_____

_____

_____

_____

_____

_____

_____

4. List the seven functions of the musculoskeletal system.

_____

_____

_____

_____

_____

_____

_____

_____

_____

_____

_____

3. Discuss changes in the musculoskeletal system due to aging

True or False

1. _____   As people age, the body loses muscle mass.

2. _____   As people age, the amount of calcium in the bones increases.

3. _____   Bones are more easily broken as people age.

4. _____   Joints become more flexible with age.

5. _____   As people age, height is gradually lost.

4. Discuss common disorders of the musculoskeletal system

Matching
Match each term below with its correct definition. Use each letter only once.

1. _____   Condition in which bones lose mass, causing them to be brittle and easily broken

2. _____   Surgical removal of an extremity

3. _____   Surgical replacement of a damaged or painful knee with artificial materials

4. _____   An artificial device that replaces a body part, such as an eye, hip, arm, leg, tooth, or heart valve

5. _____   Surgical replacement of the head of the femur and the socket it fits into where it joins the hip with artificial materials

6. _____   General term for the inflammation of the joints that can cause pain, stiffness, and swelling

7. _____   Condition in which the small sacs of fluid around the joints become inflamed

8. _____   Hereditary, progressive disease that causes muscles to weaken and stiffen, and hands and arms to twitch

9. _____   Condition that affects the synovial membrane and causes stiffness, swelling, severe pain, and deformities that can be severe and disabling

10. _____   Person feels pain in a limb or extremity that has been amputated

11. _____   Bending a body part

12. _____   Person who has had an amputation may feel warmth, itching, and tingling in the area where the limb existed

13. _____   Condition in which the cushiony cartilage that rests between the bones and pads the ends of the bones begins to slowly erode, causing pain, redness, swelling and stiffness

14. _____   A broken bone

15. ____ Method of treating fractures by keeping bones in the proper position by using weights and pulleys

(A) Amputation

(B) Arthritis

(C) Bursitis

(D) Flexion

(E) Fracture

(F) Muscular dystrophy

(G) Osteoarthritis

(H) Osteoporosis

(I) Phantom limb pain

(J) Phantom sensation

(K) Prosthesis

(L) Rheumatoid arthritis

(M) Total hip replacement

(N) Total knee replacement

(O) Traction

Short Answer

1. List eight guidelines for preventing falls.

_____

_____

_____

_____

_____

_____

_____

_____

_____

_____

_____

_____

_____

_____

_____

_____

_____

_____

_____

_____

_____

2. List five guidelines for cast care.

_____

_____

_____

_____

_____

_____

_____

_____

_____

_____

_____

_____

3. List six guidelines for care of a resident who is recovering from a total hip replacement.

_____

_____

_____

_____

_____

_____

_____

_____

_____

_____

Name: _____

4. Define partial weight-bearing (PWB), non-weight-bearing (NWB), and full weight-bearing (FWB).

_____

_____

_____

_____

_____

_____

_____

5. Describe elastic bandages

Word Search

1. Elastic bandages are also called non-_____ or self-_____ bandages.

2. Elastic bandages are used to keep _____ and _____ in place and provide _____, _____, and support for body parts.

3. These bandages are used to decrease _____ from injuries and keep _____ bags in place.

4. Elastic bandages must be wrapped snugly enough to provide the proper amount of compression and _____ but not so snugly that they interfere with _____.

5. Signs and symptoms of poor circulation include skin that is _____ to the touch and _____ marks on the skin.

s	u	d	c	i	r	c	u	l	a	t	i	o	n
u	p	w	x	n	e	v	v	g	q	g	c	o	e
p	i	l	f	d	k	l	e	n	a	j	i	k	b
p	a	q	i	e	x	t	i	i	d	s	r	u	h
o	g	k	n	n	c	e	c	r	s	k	m	m	n
r	n	l	q	t	t	q	e	e	e	o	w	v	t
t	i	n	m	a	x	s	r	h	b	t	d	f	a
d	l	y	u	t	s	p	l	d	e	h	s	n	g
b	l	w	o	i	m	c	c	a	b	f	v	f	b
l	e	o	n	o	i	t	c	e	t	o	r	p	m
i	w	g	c	n	q	c	u	d	j	s	z	p	z
g	s	j	v	m	e	n	r	e	v	n	w	f	d
t	c	f	j	h	t	k	m	p	n	n	f	e	n
o	c	t	k	i	a	q	c	k	n	f	h	i	g

Short Answer

Fill in the correct words of the "RICE" acronym for reducing pain and swelling when an injury has occurred.

R _____

I _____

C _____

E _____

22

The Nervous System

1. Review the key terms in Learning Objective 1 before completing the workbook exercises

2. Explain the structure and function of the nervous system

Fill in the Blank

1. The nervous system _____ and _____ all body functions.

2. The nervous system also _____ and _____ information from outside the body.

3. The _____ is the basic working unit of the nervous system.

4. The two main parts of the nervous system are the _____ nervous system and the _____ nervous system.

5. The right side of the brain, or right _____ controls the motor activity on the _____ side of the body, while the left side of the brain, or left _____ controls the motor activity on the _____ side of the body.

6. The peripheral nervous system consists of the _____ and _____ nerves.

7. The _____ and _____ make up the central nervous system.

8. The ear provides _____ and _____.

9. The nervous system provides _____ centers of heartbeat and respiration.

10. The sense organs are part of the nervous system. They include the _____, tongue, _____, eyes, and _____.

11. Inside the back of the eye is the _____, which contains cells that respond to light and send messages to the brain.

3. Discuss changes in the nervous system due to aging

True or False

1. ____ Weakened vision is a normal part of aging.

2. ____ Some short-term memory loss may occur with age.

3. ____ As people age, the senses normally become stronger.

4. ____ Responses and reflexes speed up with age.

5. ____ Sensitivity of nerve endings decreases with age, resulting in weakened sense of touch.

6. ____ Slight hearing loss is not a normal change of aging.

4. Discuss common disorders of the nervous system

Matching

For each of the following descriptions, write the letter of the disorder to which it refers. Use each letter only once.

1. _____ Paralysis on one side of the body

2. _____ Loss of function of the lower body and legs

3. _____ A sudden state of severe confusion due to a change in the body

4. _____ Causes a person to have recurring seizures

5. _____ Disorder of the inner ear caused by fluid build-up

6. _____ Difficulty swallowing

7. _____ Temporary or permanent state in which a person is unable to think clearly and logically

8. _____ Condition that causes the part of the retina that allows people to see detail to degenerate, destroying central vision

9. _____ Inability to understand what others are communicating through speech or written words

10. _____ An infection of the middle ear that causes pain, pressure, fever, and reduced ability to hear

11. _____ The pressure inside the eye increases, causing damage to the optic nerve

12. _____ Develops when the lens of the eye becomes cloudy, causing vision loss

13. _____ Ability to see objects that are near more clearly than distant objects

14. _____ Progressive disorder that causes loss of protective covering that protects nerves and spinal cord

15. _____ Caused by blood supply to the brain being blocked or a leaking or ruptured blood vessel within the brain

16. _____ Inability to express needs to others through speech or writing

17. _____ Tendency to ignore a weak or paralyzed side of the body

18. _____ Warning sign of CVA

19. _____ Head injury that occurs from a banging movement of the brain against the cranium

20. _____ Progressive disorder that can cause tremors and a mask-like facial expression

21. _____ Inappropriate or unprovoked emotional responses

22. _____ Loss of function of the arms, trunk, and legs

23. _____ Weakness on one side of the body

24. _____ Ability to see distant objects more clearly than objects that are near

(A) Age-related macular degeneration (AMD)

(B) Cataract

(C) Cerebrovascular accident (CVA)

(D) Concussion

(E) Confusion

(F) Delirium

(G) Dysphagia

(H) Emotional lability

(I) Epilepsy

(J) Expressive aphasia

(K) Farsightedness

(L) Glaucoma

(M) Hemiparesis

(N) Hemiplegia

(O) Meniere's disease

(P) Multiple sclerosis (MS)

(Q) Nearsightedness

(R) One-sided neglect

(S) Otitis media

(T) Paraplegia

(U) Parkinson's disease

(V) Quadriplegia

(W) Receptive aphasia

(X) Transient ischemic attack (TIA)

True or False

1. _____ Strokes that occur on the right side of the brain affect functioning on the right side of the body.

2. _____ Diminished awareness or one-sided paralysis causes a lack of sensation that increases the risk of injury.

3. _____ Residents with Parkinson's disease may do range of motion exercises to prevent contractures.

4. _____ Multiple sclerosis generally occurs in young adulthood.

5. _____ Spinal cord injuries are treated with more success if the cord is completely cut or severed.

6. _____ A cause for seizure disorders can always be determined.

7. _____ Eye drops help treat glaucoma.

Multiple Choice

1. Which of the following statements is true of a hearing aid?
   (A) To properly clean a hearing aid, it should be placed in warm water.
   (B) The battery should be turned off when it is not in use.
   (C) The volume should be turned up just before inserting it.
   (D) It needs to remain in the ear when a person is showering.

2. Which of the following statements is true of an artificial eye?
   (A) An artificial eye provides vision.
   (B) An artificial eye should be cleaned with rubbing alcohol.
   (C) An artificial eye is stored in a dry cup on a paper towel.
   (D) An artificial eye is held in place by suction.

3. When a resident has a vision impairment, a nursing assistant should:
   (A) Use the face of an imaginary clock as a guide to explain the position of items.
   (B) Keep the door partially open so that the resident can find the doorway.
   (C) Enter the room first before identifying herself, so as not to frighten the resident.
   (D) Walk behind the resident, calling out warnings when stairs and steps appear.

4. The best way that a nursing assistant can help a resident who has had a stroke is to:
   (A) Make sure the resident is constantly doing tasks in order to keep him energized.
   (B) Use short, simple sentences when communicating.
   (C) Stand on the resident's stronger side when transferring him.
   (D) Remind the resident which is his "bad leg" and which is his "good leg" so that he does not get them confused.

5. Residents who have paralysis are at a higher risk of injury from:
   (A) Heat and cold
   (B) Heart disease
   (C) Drinking too many fluids
   (D) Bowel retraining

5. Discuss dementia and related terms

Multiple Choice

1. Which of the following statements is true of dementia?
   (A) Dementia is the ability to think clearly and logically.
   (B) Dementia is the result of a normal change of aging in the brain.
   (C) Dementia is a serious loss of mental abilities that interferes with normal functioning.
   (D) Dementia is an increase in cognitive abilities.

2. The most common form of dementia is:
   (A) Parkinson's disease
   (B) AIDS
   (C) Alzheimer's disease
   (D) Excessive alcohol or drug use

3. Which of the following statements is true of dementia?
   (A) Most forms of dementia are reversible.
   (B) Dementia is the same as delirium.
   (C) Making a diagnosis of dementia is difficult.
   (D) Dementia is commonly caused by getting older.

6. Discuss Alzheimer's disease and identify its stages

Short Answer

1. Define Alzheimer's disease and briefly describe how it occurs.

   _____
   _____
   _____
   _____
   _____
   _____
   _____
   _____

2. Briefly describe what occurs in each of the seven stages of Alzheimer's disease, as developed by Barry Reisberg, M.D.

   Stage 1:

   _____
   _____
   _____
   _____

Stage 2:

_____
_____
_____
_____
_____
_____
_____
_____
_____
_____

Stage 3:

_____
_____
_____
_____
_____
_____
_____
_____
_____
_____

Stage 4:

_____
_____

_____

_____

_____

_____

_____

_____

_____

_____

_____

_____

Stage 5:

_____

_____

_____

_____

_____

_____

_____

_____

_____

_____

_____

Stage 6:

_____

_____

_____

Stage 7:

_____

_____

_____

_____

_____

_____

_____

_____

_____

_____

_____

_____

_____

_____

3. Why is it important to encourage independence in residents with Alzheimer's disease?

_____

_____

_____

Name: _____

_____

_____

_____

_____

7. List strategies for better communication with residents with Alzheimer's disease

Crossword Puzzle

Across

1. A nursing assistant should limit the times she uses this word and instead should redirect activities

4. Another name for repetitive phrasing

Down

2. These type of cues should be watched for as the ability to talk lessens

3. A nursing assistant should first _____ herself when greeting a resident with Alzheimer's disease

5. Talk about only one of these at a time using simple, short sentences

6. An example of nonverbal communication that can be used as speaking abilities decline

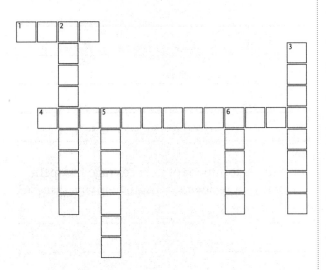

8. Identify personal attitudes helpful in caring for residents with Alzheimer's disease

Short Answer
For each of the helpful attitudes listed, write one reason why it is important.

1. Do not take it personally.

_____

_____

_____

_____

_____

_____

_____

2. Put yourself in their shoes.

_____

_____

_____

_____

_____

_____

_____

_____

3. Work with the symptoms and behaviors you see.

_____

_____

_____

_____

_____

_____

_____

_____

4. Work as a team.

_____

_____

_____

_____

_____

_____

_____

_____

5. Take care of yourself.

_____

_____

_____

_____

_____

_____

_____

_____

6. Work with family members.

_____

_____

_____

_____

_____

_____

_____

_____

7. Remember the goals of the care plan.

_____

_____

_____

_____

_____

_____

_____

_____

_____

_____

_____

9. Describe guidelines for problems with common activities of daily living (ADLs)

Short Answer
For each of the following statements, write "G" if it is a good idea for a nursing assistant to do this for a resident with Alzheimer's disease; write "B" if it is a bad idea.

1. _____ Non-slip mats, tub seats, and hand-holds should be used to ensure safety during bathing.

2. _____ The resident should always bathe at the same time every day, even if he is agitated.

3. _____ The nursing assistant should calmly explain the care she will be giving the same way every time.

4. _____ The nursing assistant should not attempt to groom the resident because the resident will not understand it.

5. ____ If the resident is incontinent, the nursing assistant should not give him fluids.

6. ____ The nursing assistant should check the resident's skin regularly for signs of irritation.

7. ____ The nursing assistant should choose clothes that are easy to put on.

8. ____ The restroom should be marked with a sign as a reminder to use it and where it is.

9. ____ For mealtime, plain plates with a simple place setting should be used.

10. ____ The nursing assistant should not encourage independence, as this leads to aggressive behavior.

11. ____ A daily calendar can be provided to encourage activities.

12. ____ The resident's weight should be monitored accurately and frequently.

13. ____ The nursing assistant should reward positive behavior with smiles, hugs, warm touches, and thank yous.

10. Describe interventions for common difficult behaviors related to Alzheimer's disease

Scenarios

Read each of the following scenarios involving residents with Alzheimer's disease and answer the questions that follow.

1. Dana is a nursing assistant who has just started working at Parkwood Care Facility. She is assigned to give Mr. Bruner, a resident with Alzheimer's disease, a bath and a back rub. When Dana meets Mr. Bruner, he gets very upset and yells at Dana to leave him alone. What can Dana do to lessen Mr. Bruner's agitation?

_____

_____

_____

_____

_____

_____

_____

_____

2. Mr. Aaronson, another resident at Parkwood, is upset because he has just found out that his daughter is moving out of the state and will not be able to visit him as often. While watching television in the common area with other residents, he gets angry at Mrs. Robinson for changing the channel. He starts shouting at her and threatens to hit her if she doesn't stop irritating him. How should Dana respond to this behavior?

_____

_____

_____

_____

_____

_____

_____

_____

3. Dana notices that one of her residents, Mr. Boyd, has seemed withdrawn lately and has not been eating as much as usual. He has lost interest in his treasured book collection and has not wanted to spend any time with his friends or family when they visit. What can Dana do?

_____

_____

_____

_____

_____
_____

4. When Dana arrives at work one morning, she gets several complaints from her residents that Mr. Bruner has been scratching his groin area in the dining room during breakfast and making the other residents at his table uncomfortable. What are some possible causes for this behavior, and how should Dana react?

_____
_____
_____
_____
_____
_____
_____

5. Ms. Stryker is a cheerful, vivacious resident with Alzheimer's disease. She loves to dress in brightly colored clothes and wear tasteful jewelry. Lately she has begun to pick up other residents' clothing and jewelry from their rooms and put them into her dresser drawer. Her family is very upset by this behavior. What should Dana tell them and how can she help?

_____
_____
_____
_____
_____
_____
_____
_____
_____

11. Discuss ways to provide activities for residents with Alzheimer's disease

True or False

1. ____ Residents with Alzheimer's disease usually do not usually enjoy participating in activities.

2. ____ Information from a resident's family should be used to plan activities for him.

3. ____ Meaningful activities for a resident with AD draw on past skills that the resident has used throughout his life.

4. ____ "Doing" activities will keep a resident with Alzheimer's focused for several hours at a time.

5. ____ If a resident loses interest in an activity, the staff should push her to continue until she is finished because it promotes a healthy self-esteem.

6. ____ Residents' families should be encouraged to participate in activities.

7. ____ Residents with AD should be discouraged from exercising.

8. ____ Each resident should be encouraged to use his or her special skills.

9. ____ Reading and playing music are good ways to provide activity for bedbound residents.

12. Describe therapies for residents with Alzheimer's disease

Matching
Use each letter only once.

1. ____ Type of therapy that promotes self-esteem, self-awareness, and socialization by having residents gather in small groups

2. ____ Type of therapy that lets people with Alzheimer's disease believe they live in the past or in imaginary circumstances

3. ____ Type of therapy that encourages people with Alzheimer's disease to remember and talk about the past

Name: _____

4. _____ Type of therapy that uses calendars, clocks, signs, and lists to help people with Alzheimer's disease remember who and where they are

(A) Reminiscence therapy

(B) Validation therapy

(C) Remotivation therapy

(D) Reality orientation

13. Discuss mental health, mental illness, and related disorders

Word Search

1. _____ _____ is a person's ability to use cognition and emotion appropriately.

2. Mental illness is a _____ that affects a person's ability to function in family, home, work, or community settings.

3. _____

_____ _____ is characterized by chronic anxiety, excessive worrying, and tension, even when there is no cause for these feelings.

4. A person who has had a traumatic experience such as being a victim of a crime or a severe accident may develop

_____ _____

_____ _____.

5. Obsessive-compulsive disorder is characterized by _____ behavior or thoughts.

6. _____ _____ disorder causes extreme self-consciousness in everyday situations and may cause a person to avoid being around other people.

7. Symptoms of _____ disorder include dizziness, rapid heartbeat, upset stomach, and a feeling of doom.

8. _____ _____ is a serious mental illness in which a feeling of overwhelming sadness makes it difficult for a person to function normally.

9. If a resident makes comments or jokes about _____ himself, report it immediately to the nurse.

10. A person with _____

_____ may have mood swings and changes in energy level and ability to function.

11. Symptoms of _____ include hallucinations, delusions, and disorganized thinking and speech.

12. A person with paranoid schizophrenia may experience delusions of

_____.

```
f  r  b  t  b  c  b  g  a  q  e  w  r  g
u  e  x  j  i  l  i  i  b  d  s  n  r  e
w  d  d  r  p  i  a  m  j  w  a  e  o  n
b  r  t  n  o  n  h  e  f  g  t  o  q  e
v  o  u  j  l  i  x  c  u  d  i  k  f  r
p  s  p  e  a  c  x  w  i  r  o  o  j  a
n  i  n  s  r  a  d  s  p  n  r  l  n  l
l  d  a  k  d  l  x  p  q  e  y  o  h  i
k  s  d  n  i  d  m  a  k  s  i  g  k  z
w  s  d  w  s  e  g  n  i  t  r  u  h  e
a  e  t  e  o  p  t  i  u  q  o  h  b  d
y  r  s  z  r  r  e  c  g  a  b  o  t  a
y  t  k  a  d  e  e  f  u  c  b  d  w  n
o  s  x  f  e  s  z  p  d  w  r  m  j  x
r  c  h  c  r  s  n  r  c  v  e  l  b  i
z  i  g  e  w  i  i  r  m  n  p  u  g  e
r  t  p  j  a  o  n  d  t  m  e  f  u  t
j  a  k  i  c  n  s  a  b  u  t  n  g  y
l  m  v  h  r  y  l  e  u  r  i  v  g  d
t  u  l  t  y  h  g  j  w  c  t  q  b  i
s  a  i  n  e  r  h  p  o  z  i  h  c  s
a  r  s  a  l  u  j  m  i  c  v  c  q  o
y  t  l  b  y  v  b  s  a  t  e  e  a  r
l  t  t  v  o  p  m  m  i  i  c  h  c  d
h  s  r  j  n  m  q  i  t  y  c  u  v  e
s  o  c  i  a  l  a  n  x  i  e  t  y  r
i  p  k  t  p  g  u  g  j  l  f  f  a  h
n  z  z  w  r  l  d  w  i  i  y  i  v  r
w  x  a  n  h  a  u  b  f  w  p  v  q  w
g  f  v  i  y  h  h  e  u  s  m  j  d  d
```

14. Discuss substance abuse and list signs of substance abuse to report

Short Answer

1. Define substance abuse.

_____

_____

_____

_____

_____

_____

2. List three risk factors for substance abuse.

_____

_____

_____

_____

_____

3. Under what circumstances is an elderly person more at risk for substance abuse?

_____

_____

_____

_____

_____

_____

23

The Endocrine System

1. Review the key terms in Learning Objective 1 before completing the workbook exercises

2. Explain the structure and function of the endocrine system

Fill in the Blank

1. Glands produce and secrete chemicals called
   _____.

2. Testosterone is produced within the
   _____.

3. The endocrine system is made up of
   _____
   in different areas of the body.

4. The endocrine system influences growth
   and _____,
   maintains blood sugar levels, and regulates
   the ability to
   _____.

5. The _____ gland, or
   master gland, controls hormone production
   of other glands.

6. During stressful situations,
   _____
   and the less potent noradrenaline increase
   the efficiency of muscle contractions,
   increase _____ rate
   and blood pressure, and increase blood
   _____ levels to provide
   extra energy.

7. The pancreas produces _____,
   which regulates the amount of glucose
   available to the cells for
   _____ .

3. Discuss changes in the endocrine system due to aging

True or False

1. _____ Menopause is a normal change of
   aging in women.

2. _____ As men age, testosterone production
   stops.

3. _____ Insulin production increases with
   age.

4. _____ As a person gets older, the body is
   less able to handle stress.

4. Discuss common disorders of the endocrine system

Matching

1. _____ Insulin reaction; a complication of
   diabetes that can be life-threatening

2. _____ Condition in which the thyroid produces too much thyroid hormone,
   causing body processes to speed up

3. _____ Glucose levels are elevated but not
   high enough to establish diagnosis of
   diabetes

4. _____ Enlarged thyroid

5. _____ Condition in which the pancreas does
   not produce insulin or does not produce enough insulin

6. _____ Causes numbness, pain, or tingling
   of the legs and/or feet and nerve
   damage over time

7. _____ Causes damage to blood vessels in
   the eyes; can cause blindness

8. ____ Most common form and milder form of diabetes

9. ____ Condition in which the body lacks thyroid hormone, causing body processes to slow down

10. ____ Form of diabetes usually diagnosed in children and young adults

(A) Diabetes

(B) Diabetic peripheral neuropathy

(C) Diabetic retinopathy

(D) Goiter

(E) Hyperthyroidism

(F) Hypoglycemia

(G) Hypothyroidism

(H) Pre-diabetes

(I) Type 1 diabetes

(J) Type 2 diabetes

5. Describe care guidelines for diabetes

True or False

1. ____ If you notice any foot problems, such as a rash or fungus on a diabetic resident's foot, wait one day before reporting it to see if it gets worse.

2. ____ Meals must be served at the same time every day for a resident with diabetes.

3. ____ If a resident with diabetes is not following her diet, report it to your supervisor.

4. ____ Always check the expiration date of test strips for blood glucose monitoring.

5. ____ As long as a sore on a diabetic resident is small (dime-sized), it does not need to be reported.

6. ____ Nursing assistants should never cut a diabetic resident's toenails.

7. ____ Exercise is unhealthy for people who have diabetes.

8. ____ Diabetic residents should go barefoot to improve circulation in the feet.

6. Discuss foot care guidelines for diabetes

Word Search

1. Diabetes weakens the _____ system, which reduces resistance to _____.

2. Poor _____ due to narrowing of _____ _____ increases the risk of infection.

3. When foot infections are not caught early, they can take months to heal. If wounds do not heal, _____ of a toe, foot, or leg may be necessary.

4. Foot care should be a part of residents' _____.

5. Avoid _____ soaps and _____ water.

6. Do not use any _____ to try to remove dirt from a toenail.

7. Use a doctor-recommended _____ or _____ on the feet, but do not use _____.

8. Remind residents not to walk around _____.

9. Notify the nurse if a resident has excessive _____ of the skin of the feet, _____ nails, or change in color of the skin or nails, especially _____.

```
f q k u k n o y c a u b l m
j b t j p g y x t y l h q k
c i r c u l a t i o n w u t
p y r x w i i j o d h o b i
v f f b j n r d h a r s h x
p u b c h f v b d i o g j x
o g n i n e k c a l b n t x
w m g n s c k u o y n i j n
d e s s o t e t z c d n c k
e v e s c i i l a a l g q k
r l c e e o t m q r a r r l
s k j g n n b a r e f o o t
r b u o m s y e t n c w e s
o k l c e q a r v u x n x y
a u f p n b f c d m p i l g
z g m c x k m u y m f m j m
d b a e c d w p g i s g a n
v k g g x a n i v t h k u n
```

24

The Immune and Lymphatic Systems and Cancer

1. Review the key terms in Learning Objective 1 before completing the workbook exercises

2. Explain the structure and function of the immune and lymphatic systems

Fill in the Blank

1. The immune system protects the body from disease-causing _____, _____, and _____.

2. _____ immunity is present at birth; _____ immunity is acquired by the body.

3. In _____ immunity, the body manufactures antibodies as a response to a foreign substance; active immunity is also acquired by a _____.

4. With _____ immunity, a person is given the antibodies needed to defend against the antigen.

5. The lymphatic system is composed of lymph, lymph vessels, lymph _____, the spleen, and the _____ gland.

6. The clear yellowish fluid that moves into the lymph system and carries disease-fighting cells, lymphocytes, is called _____.

7. A main function of the spleen is to serve as a storage shed for _____.

3. Discuss changes in the immune and lymphatic systems due to aging

True or False

1. _____ Infections may increase with age.

2. _____ Vaccines are just as effective for older people as they are for younger people.

3. _____ Antibody response speeds up with age.

4. _____ T-cells decrease in number as a person gets older.

4. Describe a common disorder of the immune system

Short Answer

1. If you had just met someone and she told you she had AIDS, how would you feel?

_____

_____

_____

_____

_____

_____

_____

_____

_____

_____

2. Resident Jeremy Lewis sees you in the hall. He looks upset. He tells you that he accidentally touched another resident with AIDS. He says that he is very worried that he will now "catch it" himself. How do you respond?

_____

_____

_____

_____

_____

_____

3. How does HIV harm the body?

_____

_____

_____

_____

_____

_____

4. List three common methods of HIV transmission.

_____

_____

_____

_____

_____

5. List four common misconceptions about HIV transmission.

_____

_____

_____

_____

_____

6. What is an opportunistic infection?

_____

_____

_____

_____

_____

_____

5. Discuss infection prevention guidelines for a resident with HIV/AIDS

Multiple Choice

1. Care for residents who have HIV or AIDS should focus on:
   (A) Helping to find a cure for HIV
   (B) Preventing visits from friends and family
   (C) Providing relief of symptoms and preventing infection
   (D) Letting residents know what new medications are available to treat the disease

2. Confidentiality is especially important to people with HIV/AIDS because:
   (A) People with HIV/AIDS who are not working in health care can be fired from their jobs.
   (B) Others may pass judgment on people with this disease.
   (C) People can be forced to be tested for HIV.
   (D) Healthcare workers with HIV/AIDS can be fined if they do not disclose their illness.

3. Which of the following is a guideline for preventing infection in residents with HIV?
   (A) Personal items should not be shared.
   (B) Sharps should be re-capped.
   (C) Nursing assistants should wear masks when talking to the residents.
   (D) Residents should be isolated from all other residents and most staff members.

6. Discuss care guidelines for a resident with HIV/AIDS

Multiple Choice

1. If a resident with AIDS has a poor appetite and is losing weight, the nursing assistant should:
   (A) Give him an over-the-counter appetite stimulant
   (B) Report to the nurse if he is not eating or enjoying his food
   (C) Let the resident know that if he does not eat, he might die
   (D) Discuss this with the resident's friends and family and see what they recommend doing

2. Which of the following statements is true of special diets for residents who have AIDS?
   (A) Residents will need to eat spicy food.
   (B) Residents will need to eat foods that are low in acid.
   (C) Residents will need to eat foods that are hard in texture.
   (D) Residents will need to eat steaming hot food.

3. Someone who has nausea and vomiting may need to:
   (A) Eat mostly dairy products
   (B) Eat small meals throughout the day
   (C) Eat one large meal at bedtime
   (D) Reduce liquid intake

4. The "BRAT" diet is helpful for:
   (A) Diarrhea
   (B) Weight gain
   (C) Nausea and vomiting
   (D) Headaches

5. Fluids are important for residents who have diarrhea because
   (A) Diarrhea causes the body to lose fluid.
   (B) Diarrhea can be prevented by drinking a lot of fluids.
   (C) Fluid intake is not important for a person who has diarrhea.
   (D) The nursing assistant will not have to offer the bedpan as often.

7. Describe cancer

Matching

1. _____ Non-cancerous

2. _____ A group of abnormally-growing cells

3. _____ Spread to other areas of the body

4. _____ Cancerous

5. _____ Type of care that works to relieve symptoms and reduce pain and suffering

6. _____ Disappearance of signs and symptoms of cancer

7. _____ Can be effective when tumors rely on specific hormones to survive and grow

8. _____ Removal of a sample of tissue for examination and diagnosis

9. _____ Cancer vaccines are one form of this

10. _____ General term used to describe a disease in which abnormal cells grow in an uncontrolled way

11. _____ Uses high-energy rays to attempt to destroy cancer cells in a specific area

12. _____ Branch of medicine that deals with study and treatment of cancer

13. _____ Goal is to remove as much of the cancer as possible

14. _____ Chemical agents or medications are administered to kill malignant cells and tissues

(A) Benign

(B) Biopsy

(C) Cancer

(D) Chemotherapy

(E) Hormone therapy

(F) Immunotherapy

(G) Malignant

(H) Metastasize

(I) Oncology

Name: _____

(J) Palliative care

(K) Radiation therapy

(L) Remission

(M) Surgery

(N) Tumor

8. Discuss care guidelines for a resident with cancer

Short Answer

For each of the following concerns for a resident with cancer, write one reason why it is important.

1. Skin care

_____

_____

_____

_____

2. Self-image

_____

_____

_____

3. Oral care

_____

_____

_____

_____

4. Pain management

_____

_____

_____

_____

5. Vital signs

_____

_____

6. Mobility

_____

_____

_____

_____

7. Nutrition

_____

_____

_____

_____

8. Bladder and bowel changes

_____

_____

_____

_____

9. Mental status and emotional needs

_____

_____

_____

_____

25
Rehabilitation and Restorative Care

1. Review the key terms in Learning Objective 1 before completing the workbook exercises

2. Discuss rehabilitation and restorative care

Short Answer

1. Define rehabilitation.

_____

_____

_____

_____

_____

_____

2. List three goals of rehabilitative care.

_____

_____

_____

_____

_____

_____

_____

_____

3. In what ways are nursing assistants vital to the rehabilitation team?

_____

_____

_____

_____

_____

3. Describe the importance of promoting independence

True or False

1. ____ Being able to perform activities of daily living by oneself is not very important.

2. ____ Dressing is one example of an activity of daily living (ADL).

3. ____ Being required to accept help with ADLs can cause a decrease in a resident's independence.

4. ____ If a resident is doing a task too slowly, a nursing assistant should offer to do it for her to help prevent the resident from being frustrated.

5. ____ Independence helps with self-esteem and can help speed recovery.

6. ____ Verbal cues are short sentences that direct a person to complete a specific step.

7. ____ Residents have a legal right to make choices about food, doctors, and how to spend their time.

4. Explain the complications of immobility and describe how exercise helps maintain health

Short Answer

For each of these body systems, write one benefit of regular activity: gastrointestinal system, urinary system, integumentary system, circulatory system, respiratory system, musculoskeletal system, nervous system, and endocrine system.

_____

_____

_____

_____

_____

_____

_____

_____

_____

_____

_____

_____

_____

_____

_____

_____

_____

_____

_____

_____

5. Describe canes, walkers, and crutches

Multiple Choice

1. How should a walker be moved?
   (A) Walker first, strong leg, then weak leg
   (B) Weak leg, strong leg, then walker
   (C) Strong leg, walker, then weak leg
   (D) Walker, weak leg, then strong leg

2. How many feet does a quad cane have?
   (A) Four
   (B) Three
   (C) Two
   (D) One

3. Which of the following walking aids is used when a resident cannot bear any weight at all on one leg?
   (A) C-cane
   (B) Quad cane
   (C) Walker
   (D) Crutches

4. Which of the following is true of using canes, walkers, and crutches?
   (A) A cane should be held on the resident's weaker side.
   (B) The resident should be wearing nonskid shoes with the laces tied.
   (C) When resident is ambulating, the nursing assistant should stay near the resident's stronger side.
   (D) When resident is ambulating, the nursing assistant should walk in front of the resident.

6. Discuss other assistive devices and orthotics

Fill in the Blank

1. Assistive or _____ devices can help people who are recovering from illness or adapting to a disability.

2. _____ is a weakness of muscles in the feet and ankles that interferes with the ability to walk normally.

3. _____ or hip wedges keep hips in proper position after hip surgery.

4. Trochanter rolls prevent the hip and leg from turning _____.

5. Handrolls help prevent finger, hand, or wrist _____.

6. Orthotic devices are devices applied externally to a limb for _____ and _____.

(F) Extension

(G) Flexion

(H) Opposition

(I) Passive range of motion (PROM)

(J) Pronation

(K) Range of motion exercises

(L) Rotation

(M) Supination

7. Discuss range of motion exercises

Matching
Use each letter only once.

1. _____ Done by resident with some help from a staff member

2. _____ Straightening a body part

3. _____ Exercises that put a joint through its full arc of motion

4. _____ Turning downward

5. _____ Moving a body part away from the midline of the body

6. _____ Done by staff without resident's help

7. _____ Turning upward

8. _____ Done by a resident alone, without help

9. _____ Touching the thumb to any other finger

10. _____ Moving a body part toward the midline of the body

11. _____ Bending backward

12. _____ Bending a body part

13. _____ Turning the joint

(A) Abduction

(B) Active assisted range of motion (AAROM)

(C) Active range of motion (AROM)

(D) Adduction

(E) Dorsiflexion

26

Subacute Care

1. Review the key terms in Learning Objective 1 before completing the workbook exercises

2. Discuss the types of residents who are in a subacute setting

Short Answer

1. What is subacute care, and where is it usually provided?

_____

_____

_____

_____

_____

_____

_____

_____

_____

2. List three conditions that might call for subacute care.

_____

_____

_____

_____

_____

_____

_____

_____

_____

_____

3. List care guidelines for pulse oximetry

True or False

1. _____ A pulse oximeter measures a person's blood oxygen level and pulse rate.

2. _____ Generally, a normal blood oxygen level is approximately 85%.

3. _____ Diseases such as COPD can lower a person's blood oxygen level.

4. _____ If the alarm on the pulse oximeter sounds, the nursing assistant should turn it off.

5. _____ The nursing assistant should report cyanotic skin or mucous membranes.

4. Describe telemetry and list care guidelines

Fill in the Blank

1. Telemetry is the application of a

_____

monitoring device.

2. The telemetry unit transmits information about the heart's _____ and _____ to a central monitoring station.

3. A portable telemetry unit attaches to a resident's _____.

Name: _____

4. Monitor _____ carefully as ordered.

5. Report if pads become _____.

6. Report to the nurse if patient has chest pain or _____, rapid _____, or shortness of _____.

5. Explain artificial airways and list care guidelines

Multiple Choice

1. An artificial airway may be needed in order to facilitate:
   (A) Ventilation
   (B) Secretions
   (C) Tachycardia
   (D) Aspiration

2. A surgically-created opening in the neck into the trachea is called a(n):
   (A) Ileostomy
   (B) Gastrostomy
   (C) Colostomy
   (D) Tracheostomy

3. When assisting a resident with an artificial airway, the nursing assistant should:
   (A) Avoid performing oral care on the resident so that the airway does not become blocked
   (B) Use other methods of communication, such as writing notes or communication boards, if resident cannot speak.
   (C) Reinsert the tubing if it falls out
   (D) Give medication to relax the resident if he bites or tugs on the tube

6. Discuss care for a resident with a tracheostomy

Crossword Puzzle

Across

3. A nursing assistant should provide this for the site around the tracheostomy

4. One position that a resident may need to be in when he has a tracheostomy

5. The cuff that attaches to the end of the tracheostomy tube in the trachea prevents this

Down

1. One reason why a tracheostomy may be necessary

2. A person with a tracheostomy may not be able to do this

3. Another name for the opening for the tracheostomy

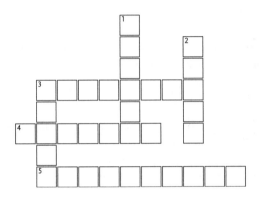

7. Describe mechanical ventilation and explain care guidelines

True or False

1. ____ A ventilator performs the process of breathing for a person who cannot breathe on his own.

2. ____ Residents on a ventilator are usually able to speak clearly, although their voice will be weaker.

3. ____ Residents on a ventilator will prefer to be left alone as much as possible.

4. ____ Residents on a ventilator are often heavily sedated.

5. ____ A resident on a ventilator needs to be positioned flat on his back at all times.

6. ____ The nursing assistant should reposition residents on a ventilator at least every two hours.

7. ____ Residents on ventilators will require one-on-one care during a power failure.

8. ____ Most residents on ventilators will show nervousness or anxiety, so it is not necessary for the nursing assistant to notify the nurse if this occurs.

8. Describe suctioning and list signs of respiratory distress

Short Answer

1. When is suctioning needed?

_____

_____

_____

_____

_____

_____

2. List four signs of respiratory distress.

_____

_____

_____

_____

_____

_____

3. List six guidelines for suctioning.

_____

_____

_____

_____

_____

_____

_____

_____

_____

_____

_____

_____

_____

_____

_____

9. Describe chest tubes and explain related care

Multiple Choice

1. Chest tubes are inserted during a _____ procedure.
   (A) Sterile
   (B) Non-sterile
   (C) Personal care
   (D) Catheterization

2. Chest tubes drain air, blood, or fluid from
   (A) The heart
   (B) The brain
   (C) The pleural cavity
   (D) The esophagus

3. Chest tubes may be required for
   (A) Vaginitis
   (B) Eczema
   (C) Nutritional deficiencies
   (D) Surgery or injuries

4. The drainage system must be
   (A) Recycled
   (B) Permanent
   (C) Airtight
   (D) Frozen

5. The drainage system must be kept _____ the level of the resident's chest.
   (A) Above
   (B) Below
   (C) Beside
   (D) At the same height as

10. Describe alternative feeding methods and related care

Matching
Use each letter only once.

1. _____ Tube placed through the skin directly into the abdomen

2. _____ Tube inserted into the nose, down the back of the throat through the esophagus, and into the stomach for feeding

3. _____ Nutrients are received intravenously, bypassing the digestive tract

4. _____ Opening in the stomach and abdomen through which PEG tube is placed

5. _____ Placed in one of the larger veins in the body when TPN is expected to be continued for a while

6. _____ Tube inserted into the mouth, down the throat, through the esophagus, and into the stomach for feeding

7. _____ Used for removal by suctioning of materials inside the body

(A) Central venous line

(B) Gastric suctioning

(C) Gastrostomy

(D) Nasogastric tube

(E) Orogastric tube

(F) Percutaneous endoscopic gastrostomy (PEG) tube

(G) Total parenteral nutrition (TPN)

11. Discuss care guidelines for dialysis

Short Answer

1. What is kidney dialysis and why is it used?

_____

_____

_____

_____

2. List five things that a nursing assistant should report to the nurse about dialysis.

_____

_____

_____

_____

_____

_____

_____

_____

_____

_____

_____

_____

27
End-of-Life Care

1. Review the key terms in Learning Objective 1 before completing the workbook exercises

2. Describe palliative care

Short Answer

1. When is palliative care given?

_____
_____
_____
_____
_____
_____
_____

2. List four goals of palliative care.

_____
_____
_____
_____
_____
_____
_____
_____
_____
_____

3. Discuss hospice care

True or False

1. ____ Hospice care is ordered by a doctor when a person has six months or less to live.

2. ____ Hospice care is generally not available on Sundays.

3. ____ Hospice care focuses on curing the resident.

4. ____ Hospice care focuses on making residents comfortable and managing their pain.

5. ____ Hospice care uses a holistic approach.

6. ____ The resident's family is not involved in hospice care.

4. Discuss the grief process and related terms

Multiple Choice

1. Mr. Anderson, a resident, talks to God about his terminal cancer. He promises to make peace with his estranged son if he is allowed to live. Which stage of dying is Mr. Anderson going through?
   (A) Denial
   (B) Anger
   (C) Bargaining
   (D) Depression
   (E) Acceptance

2. Luke, a nursing assistant, knows that his resident, Ms. Wilson, is dying. One day Ms. Wilson begins to yell at Luke, blaming him for a lack of proper care, saying, "If you had been a better caregiver, I would never have gotten sick." Luke tries to comfort her, not taking it personally because he realizes that this is the _____ stage of dying.
   (A) Denial
   (B) Anger
   (C) Bargaining
   (D) Depression
   (E) Acceptance

3. Mrs. Morris is a resident who is dying. She has an appointment with her attorney. When he visits her in her room, he says, "I just want to make sure everything is in order with your will." She thanks him nicely but tells him she has no idea why he would want to talk about that subject. Instead she wants to talk about her son. Which stage of dying is Mrs. Morris in?
   (A) Denial
   (B) Anger
   (C) Bargaining
   (D) Depression
   (E) Acceptance

4. Gwen, a nursing assistant, notices that her resident, Wes, seems a little distant. When he talks to her, he only wants to discuss the specifics of his funeral arrangements. He is very concerned about making sure his family is taken care of after he is gone. Gwen takes notes on everything he says. In which stage of dying is Wes?
   (A) Denial
   (B) Anger
   (C) Bargaining
   (D) Depression
   (E) Acceptance

5. Angelica, a nursing assistant, is worried about one of her terminally ill residents. He alternates between crying and not talking to anyone. This resident is experiencing _____.
   (A) Denial
   (B) Anger
   (C) Bargaining
   (D) Depression
   (E) Acceptance

5. Explain the dying person's rights

Short Answer
For each of the rights of a dying person listed below, write one way that a nursing assistant can honor that right.

1. The right to have visitors

   _____
   _____
   _____
   _____
   _____

2. The right to privacy

   _____
   _____
   _____
   _____
   _____

3. The right to be free from pain

   _____
   _____
   _____
   _____
   _____

4. The right to honest and accurate information

   _____
   _____
   _____
   _____

5. The right to refuse treatment

   _____
   _____

_____

_____

6. Explain how to care for a dying resident

Short Answer

Make a check mark (✓) by each suggestion below that is a good idea for a nursing assistant who is caring for a dying resident.

1. _____ Use alternative methods of communication if speech fails.

2. _____ Stop talking to a dying resident because he is probably unaware of his surroundings.

3. _____ Keep the room softly lit.

4. _____ Turn and position resident often.

5. _____ Change gowns and sheets regularly.

6. _____ Feed the resident quickly.

7. _____ Observe resident for signs of pain.

8. _____ Forcing the resident to eat and drink is a good idea because it will prolong life.

9. _____ Clean up an incontinent resident promptly.

7. Discuss factors that influence feelings about death and list ways to meet residents' individual needs

Short Answer

1. Briefly describe some ideas about death that are part of your cultural beliefs or another culture that you are familiar with.

_____

_____

_____

_____

_____

2. Have you ever experienced the death of a loved one? If so, how did you grieve?

_____

_____

_____

_____

_____

_____

_____

_____

3. List seven guidelines for meeting the psychosocial and spiritual needs of a dying resident.

_____

_____

_____

_____

_____

_____

_____

_____

_____

_____

_____

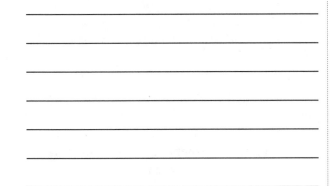

_____

_____

_____

_____

_____

_____

8. Identify common signs of approaching death

Fill in the Blank

Mark an "X" beside the signs of approaching death.

1. _____ High blood pressure

2. _____ Fever

3. _____ Cold, pale skin

4. _____ Confusion

5. _____ Healthy skin tone

6. _____ Heightened sense of touch

7. _____ Inability to speak

8. _____ Incontinence

9. _____ Perspiration

10. _____ Quick, regular breaths

9. List changes that may occur in the human body after death

Fill in the Blank

1. When death occurs, the body will not have a pulse, respiration, or _____.

2. The _____ drops, causing the mouth to stay _____.

3. _____ may be partially open with eyes in a _____.

4. Resident may have both _____ and _____ incontinence.

5. The pupils will be _____ and _____.

6. If you see any of these signs, tell the nurse so that she will _____ the death.

10. Describe ways to help family and friends deal with a resident's death

True or False

1. _____ If a family member becomes very upset after a loved one's death, it is a good idea for the nursing assistant to ask him to calm down and to stop crying.

2. _____ Family and friends may feel guilt after a loved one's death, especially if there were unresolved issues in the relationship.

3. _____ If family members seem relieved after a loved one has died, it means that they did not care for the resident very much.

4. _____ A nursing assistant should let family members and friends talk about their feelings without interrupting them.

5. _____ A nursing assistant should not let a resident's friends know that she is upset about the resident's death.

6. _____ Reassuring family and friends that they will get over the death of their loved one is helpful.

11. Describe ways to help staff members cope with a resident's death

Word Search

1. Being able to _____ is important.

2. Some facilities offer _____ to help staff with grieving.

3. Many facilities allow caregivers and residents to participate in _____ or _____ services following a death.

4. Do not be _____ because you feel grief about the death of a resident.

5. _____ and _____ are normal responses to grieving.

6. Do things that make you _____ and spend _____ time with people you love.

7. Join a special _____ for grieving.

```
b  c  r  y  i  n  g  v  h  v  z  t  v  v
s  u  p  p  o  r  t  g  r  o  u  p  s  b
a  s  h  a  m  e  d  t  m  n  k  r  e  h
d  s  b  r  n  l  a  y  s  l  y  m  k  s
n  t  x  e  b  i  m  t  a  m  s  r  m  c
e  p  h  h  f  g  r  i  e  v  e  o  n  i
s  v  v  t  p  i  r  l  t  r  y  p  w  k
s  x  m  t  g  o  l  a  q  e  s  q  m  o
d  q  p  n  m  u  u  u  e  b  r  o  p
q  q  y  e  z  s  h  q  o  t  c  s  e  k
w  f  m  m  l  n  a  r  n  i  y  z  m  x
x  o  z  e  e  f  f  i  n  g  e  o  k  y
n  m  f  v  h  f  q  p  t  f  c  z  k  a
u  x  y  a  n  d  w  p  m  t  s  b  b  m
b  k  p  e  j  w  b  n  f  h  d  i  w  i
h  p  g  r  f  c  u  s  c  y  z  a  n  r
y  e  r  e  h  p  v  m  v  g  b  k  j  a
i  l  z  b  c  j  r  n  z  k  s  f  u  q
```

12. Describe postmortem care

Short Answer

1. Define "postmortem care."

_____

_____

_____

_____

_____

_____

_____

2. What is the purpose of an autopsy?

_____

_____

_____

_____

_____

_____

3. What should a nursing assistant do after the body has been transported?

_____

_____

_____

_____

_____

_____

_____

_____

_____

_____

_____

_____

_____

_____

28

Your New Position

1. Review the key terms in Learning Objective 1 before completing the workbook exercises

2. Describe how to write a résumé and cover letter

True or False

1. _____ A person should explain his entire work history in his cover letter.

2. _____ It is best that a person's education not be listed on his résumé.

3. _____ The first step in any job search is to prepare a résumé.

4. _____ A résumé should be at least three pages long.

5. _____ A cover letter should include information on why the person is seeking the job and why he is qualified for the position.

3. Identify information that may be required for filling out a job application

Short Answer
Complete the sample job application.

Employment Application

Personal Information

Name:

Date:

Home Address:

City, State, Zip:

Home Phone:

Business Phone:

US Citizen?

If Not, Give Visa No. and Expiration Date:

Position Applying For

Title

Salary Desired:

Referred By:

Date Available:

Education

High School (Name, City, State):

Graduation Date:

Technical or Undergraduate School:

Dates Attended:

Degree Major:

References

4. Discuss proper grooming guidelines for a job interview

Short Answer
Make a check mark (✓) next to the descriptions that are appropriate for job interviews.

1. ____ Wearing rings on every finger

2. ____ Brushing your teeth beforehand

3. ____ Smoking a cigarette right before the interview to calm down

4. ____ Not wearing perfume or cologne

5. ____ Wearing jeans

6. ____ Wearing high-heeled black sandals

7. ____ Wearing artificial nails to make a better impression

8. ____ Not wearing shorts

5. List techniques for interviewing successfully

Short Answer
Make a check mark (✓) next to the behaviors that are appropriate for job interviews.

1. ____ Looking around the room while you are being interviewed

2. ____ Shaking hands firmly with the interviewer

3. ____ Practicing for the interview

4. ____ Not smiling during the interview

5. ____ Arriving 10 to 15 minutes early for the interview

6. ____ Exaggerating your accomplishments to make yourself sound more appealing

7. ____ Writing a follow-up thank-you letter

6. Describe a standard job description and list steps for following the scope of practice

Crossword Puzzle

Across

3. What a nursing assistant must do with a job description before signing it

4. An outline of what will be expected in a job

Down

1. If this is not listed in a job description, it should not be performed

2. If a nursing assistant has forgotten how to perform a procedure, she should ask this professional for a reminder

5. When a nursing assistant does something outside of her scope of practice, it can have this result for herself, a resident, or another staff member

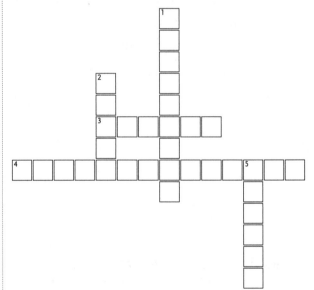

7. Identify guidelines for maintaining certification and explain the state's registry

Multiple Choice

1. What is the minimum number of hours of training a nursing assistant must complete before being employed, according to OBRA?
   (A) 50
   (B) 64
   (C) 75
   (D) 110

2. Within how many months of training must a nursing assistant usually take the state test?
   (A) 6 months
   (B) 1 year
   (C) 18 months
   (D) 24 months

3. In most states, a nursing assistant has _____ chance(s) to pass the state test.
   (A) One
   (B) Two
   (C) Three
   (D) Four

4. Which of the following is an example of information kept in the state registry for nursing assistants?
   (A) Information about investigations and hearings regarding abuse, neglect, or theft
   (B) The nursing assistant's medical records
   (C) The resident's medical records
   (D) The nursing assistant's family's medical records

8. Describe continuing education for nursing assistants

True or False

1. _____ OBRA requires that nursing assistants must have 12 hours of continuing education each year in order to keep certification current.

2. _____ The continuing education requirement for all states is the same as OBRA's.

3. _____ Subjects covered in continuing education include Residents' Rights, infection prevention, and confidentiality.

4. _____ Employers are required to provide free hepatitis B vaccines for all employees, as well as a tuberculosis test once per year.

9. Describe employee evaluations and discuss criticism

Fill in the Blank

1. An annual _____, sometimes called a performance _____ or review, is used to evaluate the performance of each employee.

2. Employees may be evaluated on overall _____, _____ resolution, and _____ effort.

3. _____ criticism is feedback that involves giving opinions about the work of others, which includes helpful suggestions for change.

4. _____ criticism is angry and negative.

5. When receiving constructive criticism, be _____ to suggestions that will help you _____ and be more _____ in your work.

6. If you are not sure how to avoid a _____ you have made, ask for suggestions.

7. Performance reviews are frequently the basis for _____.

8. A satisfactory review can increase your chances of _____ within the facility.

10. Discuss conflict resolution

Short Answer

1. What is conflict resolution?

_____

_____

_____

_____

_____

_____

_____

2. What should a nursing assistant always do when changing jobs?

_____

_____

_____

_____

11. Define "stress" and explain ways to manage stress

Matching
Use each letter only once.

1. _____ An internal or external factor or stimulus that causes stress

2. _____ Mental or physical exhaustion due to a prolonged period of stress and frustration

3. _____ Unhealthy responses to stress

4. _____ A relaxation technique for managing stress

5. _____ Appropriate people to turn to for help with stress

6. _____ Healthy ways to manage stress

7. _____ Inappropriate people to talk to about stress

8. _____ A mentally or emotionally disruptive or upsetting condition that occurs due to changes in the environment

(A) Abdominal breathing

(B) Burnout

(C) Increasing exercise, developing new hobbies, setting realistic goals

(D) Residents and residents' families

(E) Smoking, increasing caffeine in diet, taking illegal drugs

(F) Stress

(G) Stressor

(H) Supervisor, doctor, friends and family, spiritual leader

12. Describe how to be a valued member of the healthcare community

Short Answer

1. Think of two people to thank for helping you to complete your nursing assistant training course.

_____

_____

_____

_____

_____

_____

2. Think of one thing you are going to do to reward yourself for meeting this goal.

_____

_____

_____

_____

_____

_____

3. Think of one thing you will do to keep learning as you move forward in your new profession.

_____

_____

_____

Procedure Checklists

5
Infection Prevention

Washing hands

		yes	no
1.	Turns on water at the sink. Keeps clothes dry and does not let clothing touch the outside portion of the sink or counter.		
2.	Angles arms downward, with fingertips pointing down into the sink. Wets hands and wrists thoroughly.		
3.	Applies skin cleanser or soap to hands.		
4.	Rubs hands together and fingers between each other to create a lather. Lathers all surfaces of wrists, hands, and fingers, producing friction for at least 20 seconds.		
5.	Cleans nails by rubbing them in the palm of other hand.		
6.	Rinses thoroughly under running water. Rinses all surfaces of wrists, hands, and fingers. Runs water down from wrists to fingertips.		
7.	Uses a clean, dry paper towel to dry all surfaces of hands, wrists, and fingers. Disposes of towel without touching wastebasket.		
8.	Uses clean, dry paper towel to turn off the faucet. Does not contaminate hands by touching the surface of the sink or faucet.		
9.	Disposes of used paper towels in proper waste receptacle after shutting off faucet.		

_____   _____
Date Reviewed   Instructor Signature

_____   _____
Date Performed   Instructor Signature

Putting on (donning) gloves

		yes	no
1.	Washes hands.		
2.	If right-handed, slides one glove on left hand (reverses if left-handed).		
3.	Using gloved hand, slides the other hand into the second glove.		
4.	Interlaces fingers to smooth out folds and create a comfortable fit.		
5.	Checks for tears, holes, cracks, or discolored spots in the gloves. Replaces the glove if needed.		
6.	Adjusts gloves until they are pulled up over the wrist and fit correctly. If wearing a gown, pulls cuff of the gloves over the sleeves of the gown.		

_____   _____
Date Reviewed   Instructor Signature

_____   _____
Date Performed   Instructor Signature

Removing (doffing) gloves

		yes	no
1.	Touching only the outside of one glove, pulls first glove off by pulling down from the cuff toward the fingers.		
2.	As glove comes off the hand, turns it inside out.		
3.	With the fingertips of gloved hand, holds glove just removed. With ungloved hand, reaches two fingers inside the remaining glove at wrist. Does not touch any part of the outside of the glove.		

Name: _____

		yes	no
4.	Pulls down, turning this glove inside out and over the first glove as it is removed.		
5.	One glove is now held from its clean inner side. The other glove is inside it.		
6.	Drops both gloves into the proper container.		
7.	Washes hands.		

_____ _____
Date Reviewed   Instructor Signature

_____ _____
Date Performed   Instructor Signature

Putting on (donning) gown

		yes	no
1.	Washes hands.		
2.	Opens the gown. Holds it out in front of self and allows it to open/unfold. Does not shake gown or touch it to the floor. Slips arms into the sleeves and pulls the gown on.		
3.	Fastens neck opening.		
4.	Reaches behind self and pulls gown until it completely covers clothing. Secures gown at waist.		
5.	When removing gown, does not contaminate skin or clothing. Unfastens gown at neck and waist. Holds gown away from body and rolls dirty side in. Discards gown in proper container.		
6.	Puts on gloves after putting on a gown.		

_____ _____
Date Reviewed   Instructor Signature

_____ _____
Date Performed   Instructor Signature

Putting on (donning) mask and goggles

		yes	no
1.	Washes hands.		
2.	Picks up the mask by the top strings or the elastic strap. Does not touch the mask where it touches face.		
3.	Adjusts mask over nose and mouth. Ties top strings, then bottom strings.		
4.	Pinches metal strip at the top of the mask tightly around nose so that it feels snug. Fits mask snugly around face and below the chin.		
5.	Puts on goggles. Positions them over the eyes. Secures them to the head using the headband or earpieces.		
6.	Puts on gloves after putting on mask and goggles.		

_____ _____
Date Reviewed   Instructor Signature

_____ _____
Date Performed   Instructor Signature

Putting on (donning) and removing (doffing) the full set of PPE

		yes	no
	Donning:		
1.	Washes hands.		
2.	Puts on gown.		
3.	Puts on mask or respirator.		
4.	Puts on goggles or face shield.		
5.	Puts on gloves.		
	Doffing:		
1.	Removes and discards gloves.		
2.	Removes goggles or face shield.		
3.	Removes and discards gown.		
4.	Removes and discards mask or respirator.		

5.	Washes hands.		

_____ _____
Date Reviewed   Instructor Signature

_____ _____
Date Performed   Instructor Signature

7
Safety and Body Mechanics

Applying a physical tie restraint safely			
		yes	no
1.	Identifies self by name. Identifies resident. Greets resident by name.		
2.	Washes hands.		
3.	Explains procedure to resident. Speaks clearly, slowly, and directly. Maintains face-to-face contact whenever possible.		
4.	Provides for resident's privacy with a curtain, screen, or door.		
5.	Applies restraint carefully. Follows manufacturer's directions and facility policy. For each type of restraint, makes sure that it is not too tight.		
	CHEST or BELT-STYLE RESTRAINTS: Makes sure breasts or skin are not caught in the restraints.		
	VEST: Places criss-cross in the vest restraint on the front of the body.		
	MITT: Places a rolled-up washcloth or commercial hand roll in the mitt restraint.		
	WRIST/ANKLE: Makes sure restraint will not slide off the wrist or ankle.		
6.	Uses a slip knot to tie restraint. If restraint is used on a resident who is in bed, ties it to the movable part of the bed frame. Does not tie it to the side rail.		
7.	Makes resident comfortable.		

8.	Leaves call light within resident's reach.		
9.	Washes hands.		
10.	Is courteous and respectful at all times.		
11.	Reports any changes in resident to the nurse. Documents procedure using facility guidelines.		

_____ _____
Date Reviewed   Instructor Signature

_____ _____
Date Performed   Instructor Signature

8
Emergency Care, First Aid, and Disasters

Performing abdominal thrusts for the conscious person			
		yes	no
1.	Stands behind the person. Brings arms under person's arms. Wraps arms around person's waist.		
2.	Makes a fist with one hand. Places flat, thumb side of the fist against person's abdomen, above the navel but below the breastbone.		
3.	Grasps fist with other hand. Pulls both hands toward self and up (inward and upward), quickly and forcefully.		
4.	Repeats until the object is pushed out.		

_____ _____
Date Reviewed   Instructor Signature

_____ _____
Date Performed   Instructor Signature

Responding to shock			
		yes	no
1.	Notifies nurse immediately.		
2.	If controlling bleeding, puts on gloves first.		

Name: _____

3.	Has person lie down on her back. If person is bleeding from the mouth or vomiting, places her on her side (unless neck, back, or spinal cord injury is suspected).		
4.	Checks pulse and respirations; begins CPR if breathing and pulse are absent, and if trained.		
5.	Keeps person as calm and comfortable as possible. Loosens clothing or ties around neck and any belts or waist strings.		
6.	Maintains normal body temperature.		
7.	Elevates feet unless person has a head, neck, back, spinal or abdominal injury, breathing difficulties, or fractures.		
8.	Does not give person anything to eat or drink.		

_____   _____
Date Reviewed   Instructor Signature

_____   _____
Date Performed   Instructor Signature

Controlling bleeding

		yes	no
1.	Notifies nurse immediately.		
2.	Puts on gloves.		
3.	Holds thick sterile pad, clean cloth, handkerchief, or towel against the wound.		
4.	Presses down hard directly on the bleeding wound until help arrives. Does not decrease pressure. Puts additional pads over first pad if blood seeps through. Does not remove first pad.		
5.	Raises wound above level of the heart to slow down bleeding. If wound is on an arm, leg, hand, or foot, and there are no head, neck, back, spinal, or abdominal injuries or fractures, props up limb.		

6.	When bleeding is under control, secures dressing to keep it in place. Checks person for symptoms of shock. Stays with person until help arrives.		
7.	Removes gloves and washes hands thoroughly when finished.		

_____   _____
Date Reviewed   Instructor Signature

_____   _____
Date Performed   Instructor Signature

Treating burns

		yes	no
	To treat a minor burn:		
1.	Notifies nurse immediately. Puts on gloves.		
2.	Uses cool, clean water to decrease the skin temperature and prevent further injury. Does not use ice or ice water. Dampens clean towel with cool water, and places it over the burn.		
3.	Once the pain has eased, covers area with a dry, clean dressing or non-adhesive sterile bandage.		
4.	Does not use any kind of ointment, water, salve, or grease on burn.		
	For more serious burns:		
1.	If clothing has caught fire, has person stop, drop, and roll, or smothers the fire with a blanket or towel. Uses water to help put out the fire, if possible. Protects self from source of the burn.		
2.	Notifies nurse immediately. Puts on gloves.		

3.	Checks for breathing, pulse, and severe bleeding. If person is not breathing, begins rescue breathing. If the person is not breathing and has no pulse, begins CPR, if trained to do so. Does not put pillows under the head, as this may obstruct the airway.		
4.	Does not use any type of ointment, water, salve, or grease on the burn.		
5.	Does not try to pull away any clothing from burned areas. Covers burn with a clean cloth, a dry, non-adhesive sterile bandage, or a clean sheet. Applies cloth, bandage, or sheet lightly. Does not rub the burned area.		
6.	Takes steps to prevent shock.		
7.	Does not give person food or fluids.		
8.	Monitors vital signs and waits for emergency medical help.		
9.	Removes gloves and washes hands.		

_____ _____
Date Reviewed   Instructor Signature

_____ _____
Date Performed   Instructor Signature

Responding to fainting

		yes	no
1.	Notifies nurse immediately.		
2.	Has person lie down or sit down before fainting occurs.		
3.	If person is in a sitting position, has her bend forward and place her head between her knees. If the person is lying flat on her back, elevates the legs.		
4.	Loosens any tight clothing.		
5.	Has person stay in this position for at least five minutes after symptoms disappear.		

6.	Helps person get up slowly. Continues to observe her for symptoms of fainting. Uses call light if help is needed but person cannot be left alone.		

_____ _____
Date Reviewed   Instructor Signature

_____ _____
Date Performed   Instructor Signature

Responding to poisoning

		yes	no
1.	Notifies nurse immediately.		
2.	Puts on gloves. Looks for a container to help determine what person has taken or eaten. With gloves on, opens mouth and looks inside to check the mouth for chemical burns. Does not place fingers inside the mouth. Notes breath odor.		
3.	Follows any instructions from poison control.		
4.	Removes gloves and washes hands.		

_____ _____
Date Reviewed   Instructor Signature

_____ _____
Date Performed   Instructor Signature

Responding to a nosebleed

		yes	no
1.	Notifies nurse immediately.		
2.	Elevates head of the bed, or tells person to remain in a sitting position, leaning forward slightly. Offers tissues or a clean cloth to catch the blood. Does not touch blood or bloody clothes, tissues, or cloths without gloves.		

3.	Puts on gloves. Applies firm pressure over the bridge of the nose. Squeezes bridge of the nose with thumb and forefinger.		
4.	Applies pressure until the bleeding stops.		
5.	Uses cool cloth or ice wrapped in a cloth on the back of the neck, the forehead, or the upper lip to slow the flow of blood. Does not apply ice directly to skin.		
6.	Keeps person still and calm until help arrives.		
7.	Removes gloves and washes hands.		

_____   _____
Date Reviewed   Instructor Signature

_____   _____
Date Performed   Instructor Signature

Responding to vomiting

		yes	no
1.	Notifies nurse immediately.		
2.	Puts on gloves.		
3.	Places an emesis basin or wash basin under the chin. Removes basin when vomiting has stopped.		
4.	Removes soiled linens or clothes. Replaces with fresh linens or clothes.		
5.	Notes amount, color, and consistency of vomitus. Looks for blood in vomitus, blood-tinged vomitus, or medication (pills) in vomitus. Shows nurse the vomitus before discarding or if blood or pills are noted.		
6.	Flushes vomitus down the toilet and washes and stores basin.		
7.	Removes and discards gloves.		
8.	Washes hands.		
9.	Puts on fresh gloves.		

10.	Provides comfort to the person. Wipes his face and mouth. Positions him comfortably, and offers a drink of water or a sip to swish in the mouth and spit. Provides oral care.		
11.	Puts soiled linen in proper containers.		
12.	Removes and discards gloves.		
13.	Washes hands again.		
14.	Documents time, amount, color, odor, and consistency of vomitus.		

_____   _____
Date Reviewed   Instructor Signature

_____   _____
Date Performed   Instructor Signature

Responding to a myocardial infarction

		yes	no
1.	Calls or has someone call the nurse.		
2.	Places the person in a comfortable position. Encourages him to rest. Reassures person that he will not be left alone.		
3.	Loosens clothing around the person's neck.		
4.	Does not give person food or fluids.		
5.	Monitors person's breathing and pulse. If person stops breathing, performs rescue breathing. If person has no pulse, begins CPR if trained and allowed to do so.		
6.	Stays with person until help has arrived.		

_____   _____
Date Reviewed   Instructor Signature

_____   _____
Date Performed   Instructor Signature

Responding to seizures		yes	no
1.	Notes the time. Puts on gloves.		
2.	Lowers person to the floor. Cradles and protects his head. Loosens clothing to help with breathing. Attempts to turn his head to one side to lower the risk of choking.		
3.	Has someone call the nurse immediately or uses call light. Does not leave person.		
4.	Moves furniture away to prevent injury. If a pillow is nearby, places it under his head.		
5.	Does not try to stop the seizure or restrain person.		
6.	Does not force anything between person's teeth. Does not place hands in his mouth for any reason.		
7.	Does not give person food or fluids.		
8.	When the seizure is over, notes the time. Gently turns person to his left side if head, neck, or spinal injury is not suspected. Checks for adequate breathing and pulse. If the person stops breathing, performs rescue breathing. If the person has no pulse, begins CPR if trained and allowed to do so.		
9.	Reports length of the seizure and observations to the nurse.		
10.	Removes gloves and washes hands.		

_____   _____
Date Reviewed   Instructor Signature

_____   _____
Date Performed   Instructor Signature

9
Admission, Transfer, Discharge, and Physical Exams

Admitting a resident			
		yes	no
1.	Identifies self by name. Identifies resident. Greets resident by name.		
2.	Washes hands.		
3.	Explains procedure to resident. Speaks clearly, slowly, and directly. Maintains face-to-face contact whenever possible.		
4.	Provides for resident's privacy with a curtain, screen, or door.		
5.	If instructed, does these things:		
	Takes resident's height, weight, and vital signs. Documents on admission form and elsewhere per facility policy.		
	Obtains a urine specimen if required.		
	Completes the paperwork. Takes an inventory of all the personal items. Helps resident put personal items away. Labels each item if facility policy. If resident has valuables, asks nurse for instructions.		
	Fills the water pitcher with fresh water. Adds ice if requested.		
6.	When the initial portion of the admission is complete, locates family and lets them know they may return to resident's room.		
7.	Shows resident the room and bathroom. Explains how to work bed controls and call light. Points out the lights, telephone, and television and how to work them. Gives resident information on menus, dining times, and activity schedules.		

8.	Introduces resident to his roommate, if there is one. Introduces other residents and staff.		
9.	Makes resident comfortable. Removes privacy measures.		
10.	Leaves call light within resident's reach.		
11.	Washes hands.		
12.	Is courteous and respectful at all times. Asks resident if he needs anything else.		
13.	Documents procedure using facility guidelines.		

_____   _____
Date Reviewed   Instructor Signature

_____   _____
Date Performed   Instructor Signature

Measuring and recording weight of an ambulatory resident

		yes	no
1.	Identifies self by name. Identifies resident. Greets resident by name.		
2.	Washes hands.		
3.	Explains procedure to resident. Speaks clearly, slowly, and directly. Maintains face-to-face contact whenever possible.		
4.	Provides for resident's privacy with a curtain, screen, or door.		
5.	Makes sure resident is wearing non-skid shoes before walking to scale.		
6.	Starts with the scale balanced at zero.		
7.	Helps resident step onto the center of the scale, facing the scale.		
8.	Determines resident's weight.		
9.	Helps resident off the scale before recording weight.		
10.	Records the resident's weight.		

11.	Removes privacy measures.		
12.	Leaves call light within resident's reach.		
13.	Washes hands.		
14.	Is courteous and respectful at all times.		
15.	Reports any changes in resident to the nurse. Documents procedure using facility guidelines.		

_____   _____
Date Reviewed   Instructor Signature

_____   _____
Date Performed   Instructor Signature

Measuring and recording weight of a bedridden resident

		yes	no
1.	Identifies self by name. Identifies resident. Greets resident by name.		
2.	Washes hands.		
3.	Explains procedure to resident. Speaks clearly, slowly, and directly. Maintains face-to-face contact whenever possible.		
4.	Provides for resident's privacy with a curtain, screen, or door.		
5.	Adjusts bed to a safe level, usually waist high. Locks bed wheels.		
6.	Starts with scale balanced at zero.		
7.	Examines sling, straps, chains, and/or pad for any damage.		
8.	Turns linen down so that it is off the resident.		
9.	Turns resident to one side away from self (Chapter 11) or if flat pad scale is used, slides resident onto pad using a helper. If a sling is used, removes from the scale and places underneath resident without wrinkling it.		

		yes	no
10.	Turns resident back on his back and straightens sling.		
11.	Attaches sling to the scale or, if using a flat pad scale, positions resident securely on the pad.		
12.	Checks straps or other connectors, and raises the sling or the pad until the resident is clear of the bed. Secures resident before moving the scale.		
13.	For digital scales, turns them on and notes reading. With other scales, moves weights until reading is apparent. Notes weight.		
14.	Lowers resident back down on the bed. If using a sling, turns resident to both sides to remove the sling. If using a pad scale, slides resident back onto bed.		
15.	Records resident's weight.		
16.	Makes resident comfortable. Replaces bed linens.		
17.	Returns bed to lowest position. Removes privacy measures.		
18.	Leaves call light within resident's reach.		
19.	Washes hands.		
20.	Is courteous and respectful at all times.		
21.	Reports any changes in resident to the nurse. Documents procedure using facility guidelines.		

_____   _____
Date Reviewed   Instructor Signature

_____   _____
Date Performed   Instructor Signature

		yes	no
3.	Explains procedure to resident. Speaks clearly, slowly, and directly. Maintains face-to-face contact whenever possible.		
4.	Provides for resident's privacy with a curtain, screen, or door.		
5.	Helps resident to step onto scale, facing away from the scale.		
6.	Asks resident to stand straight, if possible. Helps as needed.		
7.	Pulls up measuring rod from back of scale. Lowers measuring rod until it rests flat on the resident's head.		
8.	Determines resident's height.		
9.	Helps resident off scale before recording height. Makes sure measuring rod does not hit resident in the head while helping resident off the scale.		
10.	Records height.		
11.	Removes privacy measures.		
12.	Leaves call light within resident's reach.		
13.	Washes hands.		
14.	Is courteous and respectful at all times.		
15.	Reports any changes in resident to the nurse. Documents procedure using facility guidelines.		

_____   _____
Date Reviewed   Instructor Signature

_____   _____
Date Performed   Instructor Signature

Measuring and recording height of an ambulatory resident

		yes	no
1.	Identifies self by name. Identifies resident. Greets resident by name.		
2.	Washes hands.		

Measuring and recording height of a bedridden resident

		yes	no
1.	Identifies self by name. Identifies resident. Greets resident by name.		
2.	Washes hands.		

Name: _____

3.	Explains procedure to resident. Speaks clearly, slowly, and directly. Maintains face-to-face contact whenever possible.		
4.	Provides for resident's privacy with a curtain, screen, or door.		
5.	Adjusts bed to a safe level, usually waist high. Locks bed wheels.		
6.	Turns linen down so it is off resident.		
7.	Positions resident lying straight in the supine (back) position.		
8.	Using a pencil, makes small mark on the bottom sheet at the top of the resident's head.		
9.	Makes another pencil mark at the resident's heel.		
10.	Using the tape measure, measures area between pencil marks.		
11.	Records resident's height.		
12.	Makes resident comfortable. Replaces bed linen.		
13.	Returns bed to lowest position. Removes privacy measures.		
14.	Leaves call light within resident's reach.		
15.	Washes hands.		
16.	Is courteous and respectful at all times.		
17.	Reports any changes in resident to the nurse. Documents procedure using facility guidelines.		

_____ _____
Date Reviewed   Instructor Signature

_____ _____
Date Performed   Instructor Signature

2.	Washes hands.		
3.	Explains procedure to resident. Speaks clearly, slowly, and directly. Maintains face-to-face contact whenever possible.		
4.	Provides for resident's privacy with a curtain, screen, or door.		
5.	Adjusts bed to a safe level, usually waist high. Locks bed wheels.		
6.	Positions resident lying straight in the supine (back) position.		
7.	Turns linen down and raises gown or top enough to expose only the abdomen.		
8.	Gently wraps measuring tape around resident's abdomen at the level of the navel.		
9.	Reads the number where the ends of the tape meet.		
10.	Removes tape measure. Records abdominal girth measurement.		
11.	Makes resident comfortable. Replaces clothing and bed linen.		
12.	Returns bed to lowest position. Removes privacy measures.		
13.	Leaves call light within resident's reach.		
14.	Washes hands.		
15.	Is courteous and respectful at all times.		
16.	Reports any changes in resident to the nurse. Documents procedure using facility guidelines.		

_____ _____
Date Reviewed   Instructor Signature

_____ _____
Date Performed   Instructor Signature

Measuring abdominal girth

		yes	no
1.	Identifies self by name. Identifies resident. Greets resident by name.		

Transferring a resident

		yes	no
1.	Identifies self by name. Identifies resident. Greets resident by name.		

2.	Washes hands.		
3.	Explains procedure to resident. Speaks clearly, slowly, and directly. Maintains face-to-face contact whenever possible.		
4.	Provides for resident's privacy with a curtain, screen, or door.		
5.	Collects items to be moved onto the cart, and asks another staff member to help take them to the new location.		
6.	Locks wheelchair or stretcher wheels. Helps resident into wheelchair or onto the stretcher. Takes him to the new area.		
7.	Introduces resident to new residents and staff.		
8.	Locks wheelchair or stretcher wheels. Transfers resident to the new bed, if needed.		
9.	Unpacks all belongings. Helps resident put personal items away.		
10.	Makes resident comfortable. Removes privacy measures.		
11.	Leaves call light within resident's reach.		
12.	Washes hands.		
13.	Is courteous and respectful at all times.		
14.	Reports any changes in resident to the nurse. Documents procedure using facility guidelines.		

_____   _____
Date Reviewed   Instructor Signature

_____   _____
Date Performed   Instructor Signature

3.	Explains procedure to resident. Speaks clearly, slowly, and directly. Maintains face-to-face contact whenever possible.		
4.	Provides for resident's privacy with a curtain, screen, or door.		
5.	Compares inventory list to items being packed. Asks resident to sign if all items are there.		
6.	Puts items to be taken onto the cart, and asks another staff member to help transport items to the pick-up area.		
7.	Helps resident dress in clothing of his choice. Makes sure nurse has removed all dressings, IVs, and tubes that need to be removed prior to discharge.		
8.	Locks wheelchair or stretcher wheels. Helps him safely into the wheelchair or onto stretcher.		
9.	Helps resident say his goodbyes to other residents and the staff.		
10.	Takes him to the pick-up area. Locks wheelchair or stretcher wheels. Helps resident into vehicle. Transfers personal items into the vehicle.		
11.	Says goodbye to resident.		
12.	Washes hands.		
13.	Documents procedure using facility guidelines.		

_____   _____
Date Reviewed   Instructor Signature

_____   _____
Date Performed   Instructor Signature

10
Bedmaking and Unit Care

Discharging a resident			
		yes	no
1.	Identifies self by name. Identifies resident. Greets resident by name.		
2.	Washes hands.		

Making a closed bed			
		yes	no
1.	Identifies self by name. Identifies resident. Greets resident by name.		

2.	Washes hands.		
3.	Explains procedure to resident. Speaks clearly, slowly, and directly. Maintains face-to-face contact whenever possible.		
4.	Provides for resident's privacy with a curtain, screen, or door.		
5.	Adjusts bed to a safe level, usually waist high. Locks bed wheels.		
6.	Puts on gloves.		
7.	Loosens soiled linen and rolls soiled linen (soiled side inside) from head to foot of bed. Avoids contact with skin or clothes. Places it in a hamper or linen bag. Does not place on overbed table, chair, or floor.		
8.	Removes and discards gloves. Washes hands.		
9.	Remakes bed. Places mattress pad on the bed, attaching elastic at corners as necessary.		
10.	Places bottom sheet on bed without shaking linen. If using a flat sheet with seams, places sheet with the crease in the center of the mattress. If using a fitted bottom sheet, places right-side up and tightly pulls over all four corners of the bed.		
11.	Makes hospital, or mitered, corners to keep bottom sheet wrinkle-free.		
12.	Puts on waterproof bed protector and then the draw sheet, if used. Places them in the center of the bed on the bottom sheet. Smoothes, and tightly tucks the bottom sheet and draw sheet together under the sides of bed. Moves from head of the bed to the foot of the bed.		
13.	Places top sheet over bed and centers it.		

14.	Places blanket over bed and centers it.		
15.	Places bedspread over bed and centers it.		
16.	Tucks top sheet and blanket under the foot of the bed and makes hospital corners.		
17.	Folds down the top sheet to make a cuff of about six inches over the blanket.		
18.	Takes a pillow, and with one hand, grasps clean pillowcase at the closed end. Turns it inside out over arm. Using the hand that has the pillowcase over it, grasps one narrow edge of pillow. Pulls pillowcase over it with free hand. Does the same for any other pillows. Places them at head of the bed with open end away from the door.		
19.	Returns bed to lowest position.		
20.	Leaves call light within resident's reach.		
21.	Washes hands.		
22.	Takes laundry bag or hamper to proper area.		
23.	Documents procedure using facility guidelines.		

_____   _____
Date Reviewed   Instructor Signature

_____   _____
Date Performed   Instructor Signature

Making an open bed			
		yes	no
1.	Washes hands.		
2.	Makes a closed bed.		
3.	Stands at head of bed. Grasps top sheet, blanket, and bedspread and folds them down to the foot of the bed. Then brings them back up bed to form a large cuff.		

4.	Brings cuff on the top linens to a point where it is one hand-width above the linen underneath.		
5.	Makes sure all linen is wrinkle-free.		
6.	Washes hands.		
7.	Documents procedure using facility guidelines.		

Date Reviewed _____ Instructor Signature _____

Date Performed _____ Instructor Signature _____

Making an occupied bed			
		yes	no
1.	Identifies self by name. Identifies resident. Greets resident by name.		
2.	Washes hands.		
3.	Explains procedure to resident. Speaks clearly, slowly, and directly. Maintains face-to-face contact whenever possible.		
4.	Provides for resident's privacy with a curtain, screen, or door.		
5.	Places clean linen on clean surface within reach (e.g., bedside stand, overbed table, or chair).		
6.	Adjusts bed to safe working level, usually waist high. Lowers head of bed. Locks bed wheels.		
7.	Puts on gloves.		
8.	Loosens top linen from the end of the bed on the working side.		
9.	Unfolds bath blanket over top sheet and removes the top sheet. Keeps resident covered at all times with the bath blanket.		
10.	Raises side rail (if bed has them) on far side of bed. Goes to other side of the bed. Helps resident to turn onto her side slowly, moving away from self, toward raised side rail.		
11.	Loosens bottom soiled linen, mattress pad, and protector, if present, on the working side.		
12.	Rolls bottom soiled linen toward resident and center of bed, soiled side inside. Tucks it snugly against resident's back.		
13.	Places mattress pad (if used) on the bed, attaching elastic at corners on working side.		
14.	Places clean bottom linen or fitted bottom sheet with the center crease in the center. If flat sheet is used, tucks in at top and on working side. Makes hospital corners to keep bottom sheet wrinkle-free. If fitted sheet is used, pulls two fitted corners on working side.		
15.	Smoothes bottom sheet out toward resident. Makes sure there are no wrinkles in the mattress pad. Rolls extra material toward resident. Tucks it under resident's body.		
16.	If using a waterproof bed protector, unfolds it and centers it on the bed. Smoothes it out toward resident.		
17.	If using a draw sheet, places it on bed. Tucks in on side closest to self and smoothes.		
18.	Raises side rail nearest self. Goes to the other side of bed. Lowers side rail on working side. Helps resident roll or turn onto clean bottom sheet.		
19.	Loosens soiled linen. Looks for personal items. Rolls linen from head to foot of bed, avoiding contact with skin or clothes. Does not shake soiled linen. Places it in a hamper or linen bag. Does not place on overbed table, chair, or floor.		

20.	Pulls clean linen through as quickly as possible. Starts with the mattress pad and wraps around corners. Pulls and tucks in clean bottom linen, just like the other side. Pulls and tucks in waterproof bed protector and draw sheet, if used. Makes hospital corners with bottom sheet. Finishes with bottom sheet free of wrinkles.		
21.	Places resident on his back. Keeps resident covered and comfortable, with a pillow under his head.		
22.	Unfolds top sheet. Places it over resident and centers it. Asks resident to hold the top sheet and pulls the bath blanket out from underneath. Puts it in the hamper/bag.		
23.	Places blanket over the top sheet and centers it. Places bedspread over the blanket and centers it. Tucks top sheet, blanket, and bedspread under foot of bed and makes hospital corners on each side. Loosens top linens over resident's feet.		
24.	At the top of the bed, folds down the top sheet to make a cuff of about six inches over blanket.		
25.	Holds and lifts resident's head and removes pillow. Removes soiled pillowcase by turning it inside out. Places it in hamper/bag.		
26.	Removes and discards gloves. Washes hands.		

27.	Takes a pillow, and with one hand, grasps clean pillowcase at the closed end. Turns it inside out over arm. Using the hand that has the pillowcase over it, grasps one narrow edge of pillow. Pulls pillowcase over it with free hand. Does the same for any other pillows. Places them at head of the bed with open end away from the door.		
28.	Makes sure bed is wrinkle-free. Makes resident comfortable.		
29.	Returns bed to lowest position. Returns side rails to ordered position. Removes privacy measures.		
30.	Leaves call light within resident's reach.		
31.	Is courteous and respectful at all times.		
32.	Washes hands.		
33.	Takes laundry bag or hamper to proper area.		
34.	Reports any changes in resident to the nurse. Documents procedure using facility guidelines.		

Date Reviewed   Instructor Signature

Date Performed   Instructor Signature

Making a surgical bed

		yes	no
1.	Identifies self by name. Identifies resident. Greets resident by name.		
2.	Washes hands.		
3.	Explains procedure to resident. Speaks clearly, slowly, and directly. Maintains face-to-face contact whenever possible.		
4.	Puts on gloves.		

5.	Removes all soiled linen, rolling it (soiled side inside) from head to foot of bed. Avoids contact with skin or clothes. Places it in a hamper or linen bag.		
6.	Removes and discards gloves.		
7.	Washes hands.		
8.	Makes a closed bed. Does not tuck top linens under mattress.		
9.	Folds top linens down from the head of the bed and up from the foot of the bed.		
10.	Forms a triangle with the linen. Fanfolds linen triangle into pleated layers and positions opposite the stretcher side of the bed. After fanfolding, forms a tiny tip with the end of linen triangle.		
11.	Puts on clean pillowcases. Places clean pillows on a clean surface off the bed, such as on the bedside stand or chair.		
12.	Leaves bed in its locked position. Leaves both side rails down.		
13.	Moves all furniture to make room for the stretcher.		
14.	Does not place call light on bed.		
15.	Washes hands.		
16.	Takes laundry bag or hamper to proper area.		
17.	Documents procedure using facility guidelines.		

_____   _____
Date Reviewed   Instructor Signature

_____   _____
Date Performed   Instructor Signature

11
Positioning, Moving, and Lifting

Helping a resident sit up using the arm lock			
		yes	no
1.	Identifies self by name. Identifies resident. Greets resident by name.		
2.	Washes hands.		
3.	Explains procedure to resident. Speaks clearly, slowly, and directly. Maintains face-to-face contact whenever possible.		
4.	Provides for resident's privacy with a curtain, screen, or door.		
5.	Adjusts bed to a safe level, usually waist high. Locks bed wheels.		
6.	Moves pillow to head of the bed.		
7.	Stands at side of the bed and faces the head of bed.		
8.	Spreads feet shoulder-width apart and slightly bends knees.		
9.	Places arm under resident's arm and grasps resident's shoulder. Has resident grasp caregiver's shoulder.		
10.	Reaches under resident's head and places other hand on resident's far shoulder.		
11.	At the count of three, rocks self backward and pulls resident to a sitting position. Uses pillows or a bed rest to support resident in the sitting position.		
12.	Checks resident for dizziness or weakness.		
13.	Replaces pillow. Makes resident comfortable.		
14.	Returns bed to lowest position. Removes privacy measures.		
15.	Leaves call light within resident's reach.		
16.	Washes hands.		

Name: _____

17.	Is courteous and respectful at all times.		
18.	Reports any changes in resident to the nurse. Documents procedure using facility guidelines.		

_____ _____
Date Reviewed   Instructor Signature

_____ _____
Date Performed   Instructor Signature

Assisting a resident to move up in bed

		yes	no
1.	Identifies self by name. Identifies resident. Greets resident by name.		
2.	Washes hands.		
3.	Explains procedure to resident. Speaks clearly, slowly, and directly. Maintains face-to-face contact whenever possible.		
4.	Provides for resident's privacy with a curtain, screen, or door.		
5.	Adjusts bed to a safe level, usually waist high. Locks bed wheels.		
6.	Lowers head of bed to make it flat. Moves pillow to head of bed.		
7.	If the bed has side rails, raises rail on the far side of bed.		
8.	Stands by bed with feet shoulder-width apart. Faces resident.		
9.	Places one arm under resident's shoulder blades. Places other arm under resident's thighs.		
10.	Asks resident to bend knees, brace feet on the mattress, and push feet and hands on the count of three.		
11.	Keeps back straight. At the count of three, shifts body weight to move resident while resident pushes with her feet.		

12.	Replaces pillow under resident's head.		
13.	Makes resident comfortable.		
14.	Returns bed to lowest position. Returns side rails to ordered position. Removes privacy measures.		
15.	Leaves call light within resident's reach.		
16.	Washes hands.		
17.	Is courteous and respectful at all times.		
18.	Reports any changes in resident to the nurse. Documents procedure using facility guidelines.		

_____ _____
Date Reviewed   Instructor Signature

_____ _____
Date Performed   Instructor Signature

Assisting a resident to move up in bed with assistance (using draw sheet)

		yes	no
1.	Identifies self by name. Identifies resident. Greets resident by name.		
2.	Washes hands.		
3.	Explains procedure to resident. Speaks clearly, slowly, and directly. Maintains face-to-face contact whenever possible.		
4.	Provides for resident's privacy with a curtain, screen, or door.		
5.	Adjusts bed to a safe level, usually waist high. Locks bed wheels.		
6.	Lowers head of bed to make it flat. Moves pillow to head of bed.		

7.	Stands on opposite side of bed from helper. Each person is turned slightly toward the head of the bed. Foot that is closest to the head of the bed is pointed in that direction. Stands with feet shoulder-width apart. Bends knees. Keeps back straight.		
8.	Rolls draw sheet up to resident's side. Has helper do the same on his side of the bed. Grasps sheet with palms up at resident's shoulders and hips. Has helper do the same.		
9.	Shifts weight to back foot. Has helper do the same. On the count of three, shifts weight to forward feet. Slides resident toward head of bed.		
10.	Replaces pillow under resident's head.		
11.	Makes resident comfortable. Unrolls draw sheet. Leaves it in place for next repositioning.		
12.	Returns bed to lowest position. Removes privacy measures.		
13.	Leaves call light within resident's reach.		
14.	Washes hands.		
15.	Is courteous and respectful at all times.		
16.	Reports any changes in resident to the nurse. Documents procedure using facility guidelines.		

_____ _____
Date Reviewed   Instructor Signature

_____ _____
Date Performed   Instructor Signature

Moving a resident to the side of the bed		yes	no
1.	Identifies self by name. Identifies resident. Greets resident by name.		

2.	Washes hands.		
3.	Explains procedure to resident. Speaks clearly, slowly, and directly. Maintains face-to-face contact whenever possible.		
4.	Provides for resident's privacy with a curtain, screen, or door.		
5.	Adjusts bed to a safe level, usually waist high. Locks bed wheels.		
6.	Lowers head of bed.		
7.	Stands on same side of bed to which resident is being moved.		
8.	Stands with feet shoulder-width apart. Bends knees. Keeps back straight.		
9.	Slides hands under resident's head and shoulders and moves them toward self.		
10.	Slides hands under resident's midsection and moves it toward self.		
11.	Slides hands under resident's hips and legs and moves them toward self.		
12.	Makes resident comfortable.		
13.	Returns bed to lowest position. Removes privacy measures.		
14.	Leaves call light within resident's reach.		
15.	Washes hands.		
16.	Is courteous and respectful at all times.		
17.	Reports any changes in resident to the nurse. Documents procedure using facility guidelines.		

_____ _____
Date Reviewed   Instructor Signature

_____ _____
Date Performed   Instructor Signature

Name: _____

Moving a resident to the side of the bed with assistance (using draw sheet)

		yes	no
1.	Identifies self by name. Identifies resident. Greets resident by name.		
2.	Washes hands.		
3.	Explains procedure to resident. Speaks clearly, slowly, and directly. Maintains face-to-face contact whenever possible.		
4.	Provides for resident's privacy with a curtain, screen, or door.		
5.	Adjusts bed to a safe level, usually waist high. Locks bed wheels.		
6.	Lowers head of bed. Moves pillow to head of bed.		
7.	Stands on opposite side of bed from helper, facing helper. Stands up straight, facing side of bed, with feet shoulder-width apart. Points feet toward side of bed. Bends knees.		
8.	Rolls draw sheet up to resident's side. Has helper do the same on his side of the bed. Grasps sheet with palms up at resident's shoulders and hips. Has helper do the same.		
9.	On the count of three, slides resident toward side of bed, with weight equal on each foot.		
10.	Replaces pillow under resident's head.		
11.	Makes resident comfortable. Unrolls draw sheet. Leaves it in place for the next repositioning.		
12.	Returns bed to lowest position. Removes privacy measures.		
13.	Leaves call light within resident's reach.		
14.	Washes hands.		

15.	Is courteous and respectful at all times.		
16.	Reports any changes in resident to the nurse. Documents procedure using facility guidelines.		

_____ _____
Date Reviewed   Instructor Signature

_____ _____
Date Performed   Instructor Signature

Turning a resident away from you

		yes	no
1.	Identifies self by name. Identifies resident. Greets resident by name.		
2.	Washes hands.		
3.	Explains procedure to resident. Speaks clearly, slowly, and directly. Maintains face-to-face contact whenever possible.		
4.	Provides for resident's privacy with a curtain, screen, or door.		
5.	Adjusts bed to a safe level, usually waist high. Locks bed wheels.		
6.	Lowers head of bed.		
7.	Stands on side of bed opposite to where resident will be turned. Raises far side rail. Lowers side rail nearest self if it is up.		
8.	Moves resident to side of bed nearest self, using previous procedure.		
9.	Crosses resident's arm over his or her chest. Moves arm on side resident is being turned to out of the way. Crosses leg nearest self over the far leg.		
10.	Stands with feet shoulder-width apart. Bends knees.		
11.	Places one hand on resident's shoulder. Places other hand on resident's nearest hip.		

12.	Pushes onto side as one unit, toward the other side of bed (toward raised side rail). Shifts weight from back leg to front leg. Makes sure resident's face is not covered by the pillow.		
13.	Positions resident properly in good alignment:		
	• Head supported by pillow		
	• Shoulder adjusted so resident is not lying on arm		
	• Top arm supported by pillow		
	• Back supported by supportive device		
	• Hips properly aligned		
	• Top knee flexed		
	• Supportive device between legs with top knee flexed; knee and ankle supported		
14.	Covers resident with top linens. Makes resident comfortable.		
15.	Returns bed to lowest position. Returns side rails to ordered position. Removes privacy measures.		
16.	Leaves call light within resident's reach.		
17.	Washes hands.		
18.	Is courteous and respectful at all times.		
19.	Reports any changes in resident to the nurse. Documents procedure using facility guidelines.		

_____   _____
Date Reviewed   Instructor Signature

_____   _____
Date Performed   Instructor Signature

Turning a resident toward you		yes	no
1.	Identifies self by name. Identifies resident. Greets resident by name.		
2.	Washes hands.		

3.	Explains procedure to resident. Speaks clearly, slowly, and directly. Maintains face-to-face contact whenever possible.		
4.	Provides for resident's privacy with a curtain, screen, or door.		
5.	Adjusts bed to a safe level, usually waist high. Locks bed wheels.		
6.	Lowers head of bed.		
7.	Stands on side of bed opposite to where resident will be turned. Raises far side rail. Lowers side rail nearest self if it is up.		
8.	Moves resident to side of bed nearest self using previous procedure.		
9.	Crosses resident's arm over his or her chest. Moves arm on side resident is being turned to out of the way. Crosses leg furthest from self over the near leg.		
10.	Stands with feet shoulder-width apart. Bends knees.		
11.	Places one hand on resident's far shoulder. Places other hand on the resident's far hip.		
12.	Rolls resident toward self. Makes sure resident's face is not covered by pillow.		
13.	Positions resident properly in good alignment:		
	• Head supported by pillow		
	• Shoulder adjusted so resident is not lying on arm		
	• Top arm supported by pillow		
	• Back supported by supportive device		
	• Hips properly aligned		
	• Top knee flexed		
	• Supportive device between legs with top knee flexed; knee and ankle supported		
14.	Covers resident with top linens. Makes resident comfortable.		

15.	Returns bed to lowest position. Returns side rails to ordered position. Removes privacy measures.		
16.	Leaves call light within resident's reach.		
17.	Washes hands.		
18.	Is courteous and respectful at all times.		
19.	Reports any changes in resident to the nurse. Documents procedure using facility guidelines.		

_____   _____
Date Reviewed   Instructor Signature

_____   _____
Date Performed   Instructor Signature

Logrolling a resident with assistance

		yes	no
1.	Identifies self by name. Identifies resident. Greets resident by name.		
2.	Washes hands.		
3.	Explains procedure to resident. Speaks clearly, slowly, and directly. Maintains face-to-face contact whenever possible.		
4.	Provides for resident's privacy with a curtain, screen, or door.		
5.	Adjusts bed to a safe level, usually waist high. Locks bed wheels.		
6.	Lowers head of bed.		
7.	With both workers on same side of bed, stands at resident's head and shoulders. Other worker stands near resident's midsection.		
8.	Places pillow under resident's head to support neck during move.		
9.	Places resident's arms across his or her chest. Places pillow between the knees.		

10.	Stands with feet shoulder-width apart. Bends knees.		
11.	Grasps draw sheet on the far side.		
12.	On the count of three, rolls resident toward self, turning as a unit.		
13.	Repositions resident comfortably in good alignment. Places pillow under head. Covers resident with top linens.		
14.	Returns bed to lowest position. Removes privacy measures.		
15.	Leaves call light within resident's reach.		
16.	Washes hands.		
17.	Is courteous and respectful at all times.		
18.	Reports any changes in resident to the nurse. Documents procedure using facility guidelines.		

_____   _____
Date Reviewed   Instructor Signature

_____   _____
Date Performed   Instructor Signature

Assisting a resident to sit up on side of bed: dangling

		yes	no
1.	Identifies self by name. Identifies resident. Greets resident by name.		
2.	Washes hands.		
3.	Explains procedure to resident. Speaks clearly, slowly, and directly. Maintains face-to-face contact whenever possible.		
4.	Provides for resident's privacy with a curtain, screen, or door.		
5.	Adjusts bed to a safe level, usually waist high. Locks bed wheels.		
6.	Raises head of bed to sitting position. Folds linen to the foot of the bed.		

7.	Stands at side of bed with feet shoulder-width apart. Bends knees. Keeps back straight. Helps resident slowly move toward self.		
8.	Places one arm under resident's shoulder blades. Places other arm under resident's thighs.		
9.	On the count of three, turns resident into sitting position with legs dangling over the side of bed.		
10.	Asks resident to sit up straight and push both fists into the edge of mattress. Assists resident to put on non-skid shoes, if she is going to get out of bed.		
11.	Has resident dangle as long as ordered.		
12.	Takes vital signs as ordered.		
13.	Removes shoes.		
14.	Assists resident back into bed. Places one arm around resident's shoulders. Places other arm under resident's knees. Moves resident's legs onto bed.		
15.	Makes resident comfortable. Covers resident with top linens. Replaces pillow under resident's head.		
16.	Returns bed to lowest position. Removes privacy measures.		
17.	Leaves call light within resident's reach.		
18.	Washes hands.		
19.	Is courteous and respectful at all times.		
20.	Reports any changes in resident to the nurse. Documents procedure using facility guidelines.		

_____   _____
Date Reviewed   Instructor Signature

_____   _____
Date Performed   Instructor Signature

Applying a transfer belt

		yes	no
1.	Identifies self by name. Identifies resident. Greets resident by name.		
2.	Washes hands.		
3.	Explains procedure to resident. Speaks clearly, slowly, and directly. Maintains face-to-face contact whenever possible.		
4.	Provides for resident's privacy with a curtain, screen, or door.		
5.	Adjusts bed to a safe level, usually waist high. Locks bed wheels.		
6.	Supporting the back and hips, assists resident to a sitting position with feet flat on the floor.		
7.	Puts on and properly fastens non-skid footwear on resident.		
8.	Places belt over resident's clothing below the rib cage and above the waist. Does not put it over bare skin.		
9.	Tightens buckle until it is snug. Leaves enough room to insert three fingers into the belt.		
10.	Checks to make sure that breasts are not caught under belt.		
11.	Positions buckle slightly off-center in the front or back for comfort.		

_____   _____
Date Reviewed   Instructor Signature

_____   _____
Date Performed   Instructor Signature

Transferring a resident from bed to a chair or wheelchair

		yes	no
1.	Identifies self by name. Identifies resident. Greets resident by name.		

Name: _____

2.	Washes hands.		
3.	Explains procedure to resident. Speaks clearly, slowly, and directly. Maintains face-to-face contact whenever possible.		
4.	Provides for resident's privacy with a curtain, screen, or door.		
5.	Removes wheelchair footrests close to the bed.		
6.	Places wheelchair near head of the bed with arm of wheelchair almost touching the bed. Wheelchair is facing the foot of the bed. Places wheelchair on resident's stronger side.		
7.	Locks wheelchair wheels.		
8.	Raises head of bed. Adjusts bed level so that height of bed is equal to or slightly higher than the chair. Locks bed wheels.		
9.	Assists resident to a sitting position with feet flat on the floor.		
10.	Puts non-skid footwear on resident and fastens securely.		
11.	**With transfer belt**:		
a.	Stands in front of resident.		
b.	Stands with feet about shoulder-width apart. Bends knees. Keeps back straight.		
c.	Places belt below the rib cage and above the waist. Does not put it over bare skin. Grasps belt securely on both sides.		
	Without transfer belt:		
a.	Stands in front of resident.		
b.	Stands with feet about shoulder-width apart. Bends knees. Keeps back straight.		
c.	Places arms around resident's torso under the arms, but not in the armpits.		
12.	Provides instructions to allow resident to help with transfer.		

13.	With legs, braces resident's lower legs to prevent slipping.		
14.	On the count of three, helps resident to stand.		
15.	Tells resident to take small steps in the direction of the chair while turning her back toward the chair.		
16.	Asks resident to put hands on wheelchair armrests, if able. When the resident's legs touch the back of the chair, helps her lower herself into chair.		
17.	Repositions resident with hips touching back of wheelchair. Removes transfer belt, if used.		
18.	Attaches footrests. Places resident's feet on footrests. Checks that resident is in good alignment.		
19.	Makes resident comfortable.		
20.	Removes privacy measures.		
21.	Leaves call light within resident's reach.		
22.	Washes hands.		
23.	Is courteous and respectful at all times.		
24.	Reports any changes in resident to the nurse. Documents procedure using facility guidelines.		
	To transfer back to bed from a wheelchair, follow these steps:		
1.	Performs steps 1 through 7 above.		
2.	Adjusts bed level to a low position, with height of bed equal to or slightly lower than the chair. Locks bed wheels.		
3.	Performs steps 11 through 14 above.		
4.	Helps resident pivot to bed with back of resident's legs against bed. When resident feels the bed, he slowly sits down on the side of the bed.		

5.	Makes resident comfortable. Removes transfer belt, if used.		
6.	Returns bed to lowest position. Removes privacy measures.		
7.	Leaves call light within resident's reach.		
8.	Washes hands.		
9.	Is courteous and respectful at all times.		
10.	Reports any changes in resident to the nurse. Documents procedure using facility guidelines.		

_____   _____
Date Reviewed   Instructor Signature

_____   _____
Date Performed   Instructor Signature

Transferring a resident from bed to stretcher with assistance

		yes	no
1.	Identifies self by name. Identifies resident. Greets resident by name.		
2.	Washes hands.		
3.	Explains procedure to resident. Speaks clearly, slowly, and directly. Maintains face-to-face contact whenever possible.		
4.	Provides for resident's privacy with a curtain, screen, or door.		
5.	Lowers head of bed so that it is flat. Locks bed wheels.		
6.	Folds linens to foot of the bed. Covers resident with bath blanket.		
7.	Moves resident to the side of bed.		
8.	Places stretcher solidly against bed, with bed height equal to or slightly above height of stretcher. Locks stretcher wheels. Moves stretcher safety belts out of the way.		
9.	Two workers are on the side of the bed opposite the stretcher. Two more workers are on the other side of the stretcher.		
10.	Each worker rolls up the sides of the draw sheet and prepares to move resident.		
11.	On the count of three, lifts and moves resident to stretcher.		
12.	Raises head of stretcher or places a pillow under resident's head.		
13.	Places safety straps across resident. Raises side rails on stretcher.		
14.	Unlocks stretcher's wheels. Takes resident to proper site. Stays with the resident until another team member takes over responsibility of the resident.		
15.	Washes hands.		
16.	Is courteous and respectful at all times.		
17.	Reports any changes in resident to the nurse. Documents procedure using facility guidelines.		
	To transfer back to bed from stretcher:		
	The bed height should be equal to or slightly below the stretcher when transferring the resident back to bed.		

_____   _____
Date Reviewed   Instructor Signature

_____   _____
Date Performed   Instructor Signature

Transferring a resident using a mechanical lift with assistance

		yes	no
1.	Identifies self by name. Identifies resident. Greets resident by name.		

2.	Washes hands.		
3.	Explains procedure to resident. Speaks clearly, slowly, and directly. Maintains face-to-face contact whenever possible.		
4.	Provides for resident's privacy with a curtain, screen, or door.		
5.	Locks bed wheels.		
6.	Removes wheelchair footrests close to the bed. Positions wheelchair next to bed. Locks wheelchair brakes.		
7.	Raises farthest side rail. Lowers side rail nearest self if it is up. Helps resident turn to one side of the bed, away from self. Pads the sling where the neck will rest with a washcloth for resident's comfort. Positions sling under the resident, with the edge next to the resident's back. Fanfolds if possible. Makes bottom of sling even with the resident's knees. Helps resident roll to his opposite side. Spreads out fanfolded edge of the sling, then rolls him back to the middle of the bed.		
8.	Rolls mechanical lift to bedside. Makes sure the base is opened to its widest point. Pushes base of the lift under bed. Locks lift wheels.		
9.	Places overhead bar directly over resident.		
10.	With the resident lying on his back, attaches one set of straps to each side of the sling. Attaches one set of straps to overhead bar. Has co-worker support the resident at the head, shoulders, and knees while being lifted. Makes sure all straps are connected properly.		

11.	Following manufacturer's instructions, raises resident two inches above the bed. Pauses a moment for the resident to regain stability or balance. Unlocks lift wheels.		
12.	Has co-worker support and guide resident's body until resident is positioned over the chair or wheelchair.		
13.	Lowers resident into chair or wheelchair. Pushes down gently on resident's knees to help resident into a sitting position.		
14.	Undoes straps from overhead bar. Leaves sling in place for transfer back to bed.		
15.	Makes sure resident is seated comfortably and correctly in the chair or wheelchair. Puts non-skid footwear on resident and fastens. Replaces footrests.		
16.	Removes privacy measures.		
17.	Leaves call light within resident's reach.		
18.	Washes hands.		
19.	Is courteous and respectful at all times.		
20.	Reports any changes in resident to the nurse. Documents procedure using facility guidelines.		

_____ _____
Date Reviewed   Instructor Signature

_____ _____
Date Performed   Instructor Signature

Transferring a resident onto and off a toilet			
		yes	no
1.	Identifies self by name. Identifies resident. Greets resident by name.		
2.	Washes hands.		

3.	Explains procedure to resident. Speaks clearly, slowly, and directly. Maintains face-to-face contact whenever possible.		
4.	Provides for resident's privacy with a curtain, screen, or door.		
5.	Positions wheelchair at a right angle to the toilet to face hand bar/wall rail. Places wheelchair on resident's stronger side.		
6.	Removes wheelchair footrests. Locks wheels. Puts non-skid footwear on resident. Fastens securely.		
7.	Puts on gloves. Asks resident to push against the armrests of the wheelchair and stand, reaching for and grasping the hand bar with her stronger arm. Moves wheelchair out of the way.		
8.	Asks resident to pivot her feet and back up so that she can feel the front of the toilet with the back of her legs.		
9.	Helps resident to pull down underwear and pants.		
10.	Helps resident to slowly sit down onto the toilet. Allows for privacy unless resident cannot be left alone. Closes bathroom door. Stays near the door until resident is finished.		
11.	When the resident is finished, assists with perineal care as necessary. Asks her to stand and reach for the hand bar.		
12.	Uses toilet tissue or damp cloth to clean the resident. Makes sure she is clean and dry before pulling up clothing. Removes and discards gloves.		
13.	Helps resident to the sink to wash hands.		
14.	Washes hands.		

15.	Helps resident back into wheelchair. Makes sure the resident is seated comfortably and correctly in the wheelchair. Replaces footrests.		
16.	Helps resident to leave the bathroom.		
17.	Leaves call light within resident's reach.		
18.	Washes hands.		
19.	Is courteous and respectful at all times.		
20.	Reports any changes in resident to the nurse. Documents procedure using facility guidelines.		

_____ _____
Date Reviewed   Instructor Signature

_____ _____
Date Performed   Instructor Signature

Transferring a resident into a vehicle

		yes	no
1.	Identifies self by name. Identifies resident. Greets resident by name.		
2.	Washes hands.		
3.	Explains procedure to resident. Speaks clearly, slowly, and directly. Maintains face-to-face contact whenever possible.		
4.	Places wheelchair close to the vehicle at a 45-degree angle. Opens door on the resident's stronger side, if possible.		
5.	Locks wheelchair.		
6.	Asks resident to push against arm rests of the wheelchair and stand.		
7.	Asks resident to stand, grasp the vehicle or dashboard, and pivot his foot so the side of the seat touches the back of the legs.		

Name: _____

		yes	no
8.	Has resident sit in the seat and lift one leg, and then the other, into the vehicle.		
9.	Positions resident comfortably in the vehicle. Helps fasten seat belt.		
10.	Has co-worker place belongings in vehicle. Shuts the door(s).		
11.	Returns wheelchair to the appropriate place for cleaning.		
12.	Washes hands.		
13.	Documents procedure using facility guidelines.		

_____   _____
Date Reviewed   Instructor Signature

_____   _____
Date Performed   Instructor Signature

Assisting a resident to ambulate

		yes	no
1.	Identifies self by name. Identifies resident. Greets resident by name.		
2.	Washes hands.		
3.	Explains procedure to resident. Speaks clearly, slowly, and directly. Maintains face-to-face contact whenever possible.		
4.	Provides for resident's privacy with a curtain, screen, or door.		
5.	Adjusts bed to lowest position so that resident's feet are flat on the floor. Locks bed wheels.		
6.	Puts non-skid footwear on resident. Fastens securely.		
7.	Helps resident move to a dangling position, as described in earlier procedure.		
8.	Stands in front of and faces resident. Stands with feet shoulder-width apart. Bends knees. Keeps back straight.		

9.	*With gait belt*: Places belt below the rib cage and above the waist. Does not put it over bare skin. Grasps belt on both sides.		
	Without gait belt: Places arms around resident's torso under the arms, but not in the armpits.		
10.	With legs, braces resident's lower legs to prevent slipping.		
11.	On the count of three, slowly helps resident to stand.		
12.	*With gait belt*: Walks slightly behind and to one side of resident for the full distance, while holding onto the gait belt. If the resident has a weaker side, stands on the weaker side. Asks resident to look forward, not down at floor, during ambulation.		
	Without gait belt: Walks slightly behind and to one side of resident for the full distance. Supports resident's back with arm. Asks resident to look forward, not down at floor, during ambulation.		
13.	After ambulation, makes resident comfortable. Removes gait belt, if used.		
14.	Returns bed to lowest position. Removes privacy measures.		
15.	Leaves call light within resident's reach.		
16.	Washes hands.		
17.	Is courteous and respectful at all times.		
18.	Reports any changes in resident to the nurse. Documents procedure using facility guidelines.		

_____   _____
Date Reviewed   Instructor Signature

_____   _____
Date Performed   Instructor Signature

12
Personal Care

Giving a complete bed bath		yes	no
1.	Identifies self by name. Identifies resident. Greets resident by name.		
2.	Washes hands.		
3.	Explains procedure to resident. Speaks clearly, slowly, and directly. Maintains face-to-face contact whenever possible.		
4.	Provides for resident's privacy with a curtain, screen, or door.		
5.	Adjusts bed to a safe level, usually waist high. Locks bed wheels.		
6.	Places a bath blanket or towel over resident. Asks him to hold onto it as bedding is folded back. Removes gown, while keeping resident covered with bath blanket.		
7.	Fills basin with warm water. Tests water temperature with thermometer or wrist and ensures it is safe. Has resident check water temperature. Adjusts if necessary. Changes water when it becomes too cool, soapy, or dirty.		
8.	Puts on gloves.		
9.	Asks resident to participate in washing.		
10.	Uncovers only one part of body at a time. Places towel under the body part being washed.		
11.	Washes, rinses, and dries one part of the body at a time. Starts at head. Works down, and completes the front first. When washing, uses a clean area of the washcloth for each stroke.		

Eyes, Face, Ears, Neck: Washes face with wet washcloth (no soap). Begins with the eye farther away from self. Washes inner area to outer area. Uses a different area of the washcloth for each eye. Washes face from the middle outward. Washes ears and behind the ears and the neck. Rinses and pats dry with blotting motion.			
Arms and Axillae: Removes one arm from under the towel. With a soapy washcloth, washes upper arm and underarm. Uses long strokes from the shoulder to the wrist. Rinses and pats dry. Repeats for the other arm.			
Hands: Washes one hand in a basin. Cleans under the nails with an orangewood stick or nail brush. Rinses and pats dry. Makes sure to dry between the fingers. Gives nail care. Repeats for the other hand. Puts lotion on the resident's elbows and hands if ordered.			
Chest: Places towel across resident's chest. Pulls bath blanket down to the waist. Lifts the towel only enough to wash the chest. Rinses it and pats dry. For a female resident, washes, rinses, and dries breasts and under breasts. Checks skin in this area for signs of irritation.			
Abdomen: Keeps towel across chest. Folds bath blanket down so that it still covers the genital area. Washes abdomen, rinses, and pats dry. Covers with towel. Pulls bath blanket up to the resident's chin. Removes towel.			

Name: _____

	Legs and Feet: Exposes one leg. Places a towel under it. Washes the thigh. Uses long, downward strokes. Rinses and pats dry. Does the same from the knee to the ankle.		
	Places another towel under the foot. Moves basin to the towel. Places foot into basin. Washes foot and between the toes. Rinses foot and pats dry. Dries between toes. Gives nail care if it has been assigned. Applies lotion to the foot if ordered, especially at the heels. Does not apply lotion between the toes. Repeats steps for the other leg and foot.		
	Back: Helps resident move to center of the bed. Asks resident to turn onto his side so his back is facing self. If the bed has rails, raises rail on the far side for safety. Folds blanket away from the back. Places a towel lengthwise next to the back. Washes the back, neck, and buttocks with long, downward strokes. Rinses and pats dry. Applies lotion if ordered.		
12.	Places towel under the buttocks and upper thighs. Helps the resident turn onto his back. If the resident is able to wash his or her perineal area, places a basin of clean, warm water and a washcloth and towel within reach. Hands items to the resident as needed. Removes and discards gloves if asked to leave the room. Washes hands. Leaves supplies and the call light within reach. If the resident has a urinary catheter in place, reminds him not to pull on it.		

13.	If the resident cannot provide perineal care, removes and discards gloves. Washes hands. Puts on clean gloves.		
14.	**Perineal area and buttocks**: Changes bath water. Washes, rinses, and dries perineal area. Works from front to back (clean to dirty).		
	For a female resident: Uses water and a small amount of soap, and cleans from front to back. Uses single strokes. Uses a clean area of washcloth or clean washcloth for each stroke.		
	Separates the labia majora and cleans from front to back on one side with a clean washcloth, using a single stroke. Using a clean area of washcloth, cleans the other side. Cleans the perineum (area between genitals and anus) last with a front to back motion. Rinses the area thoroughly in the same way. Makes sure all soap is removed.		
	Dries entire perineal area. Moves from front to back. Asks resident to turn on her side. Washes, rinses, and dries buttocks and anal area. Cleans anal area without contaminating the perineal area.		
	For a male resident: If the resident is uncircumcised, pulls back the foreskin first. Pushes skin toward the base of penis. Holds penis by the shaft. Washes in a circular motion from the tip down to the base. Uses clean area of washcloth or clean washcloth for each stroke.		

Name: _____

	Thoroughly rinses the penis. If resident is uncircumcised, returns foreskin to normal position. Then washes scrotum and groin. Rinses thoroughly and pats dry. Asks resident to turn on his side. Washes, rinses, and dries buttocks and anal area. Cleans anal area without contaminating the perineal area.		
15.	Empties, rinses, and dries bath basin. Places basin in designated dirty supply area or returns to storage, depending on policy.		
16.	Places soiled clothing and linens in proper containers.		
17.	Removes and discards gloves.		
18.	Washes hands.		
19.	Provides deodorant.		
20.	Puts clean gown or clothes on resident. Assists with brushing or combing resident's hair.		
21.	Removes bath blanket. Replaces bedding. Makes resident comfortable.		
22.	Returns bed to lowest position. Removes privacy measures.		
23.	Leaves call light within resident's reach.		
24.	Washes hands.		
25.	Is courteous and respectful at all times.		
26.	Reports any changes in resident to the nurse. Documents procedure using facility guidelines.		

_____   _____
Date Reviewed   Instructor Signature

_____   _____
Date Performed   Instructor Signature

Shampooing a resident's hair in bed			
		yes	no
1.	Identifies self by name. Identifies resident. Greets resident by name.		
2.	Washes hands.		
3.	Explains procedure to resident. Speaks clearly, slowly, and directly. Maintains face-to-face contact whenever possible.		
4.	Provides for resident's privacy with a curtain, screen, or door.		
5.	Adjusts bed to a safe level, usually waist high. Locks bed wheels.		
6.	Lowers head of bed. Removes pillow.		
7.	Tests water temperature with thermometer or wrist. Ensures it is safe. Has resident check water temperature. Adjusts if necessary.		
8.	Puts on gloves.		
9.	Places waterproof pad under resident's head and shoulders. Covers resident with the bath blanket. Folds back the top sheet and regular blankets.		
10.	Places trough under resident's head. Connects trough to catch basin. Places one towel across the resident's shoulders.		
11.	Protects resident's eyes with dry washcloth.		
12.	Uses pitcher or attachment to wet hair thoroughly. Applies a small amount of shampoo, usually the size of a quarter.		
13.	Lathers and massages scalp with fingertips. Uses a circular motion from front to back.		
14.	Rinses hair until water runs clear. Applies conditioner. Rinses hair thoroughly to prevent the scalp from getting dry and itchy.		

		yes	no
15.	Wraps resident's hair in a clean towel. Dries his face with washcloth used to protect eyes. Gently rubs the scalp and hair with the towel.		
16.	Removes trough and waterproof covering.		
17.	Empties, rinses, and wipes bath basin/pitcher. Returns to proper storage.		
18.	Places soiled linen in proper container.		
19.	Removes and discards gloves. Washes hands.		
20.	Raises head of bed.		
21.	Dries and combs resident's hair as he or she prefers. Returns hair dryer and comb/brush to proper storage.		
22.	Makes resident comfortable.		
23.	Returns bed to lowest position. Removes privacy measures.		
24.	Leaves call light within resident's reach.		
25.	Washes hands.		
26.	Is courteous and respectful at all times.		
27.	Reports any changes in resident to the nurse. Documents procedure using facility guidelines.		

_____   _____
Date Reviewed   Instructor Signature

_____   _____
Date Performed   Instructor Signature

Giving a shower or tub bath

		yes	no
1.	Washes hands.		
2.	Places equipment in shower or tub room. Puts on gloves. Cleans shower or tub area and shower chair.		
3.	Removes and discards gloves.		
4.	Washes hands.		
5.	Goes to resident's room. Identifies self by name. Identifies the resident. Greets the resident by name.		
6.	Explains procedure to resident. Speaks clearly, slowly, and directly. Maintains face-to-face contact whenever possible.		
7.	Provides for resident's privacy with a curtain, screen, or door.		
8.	Helps resident to put on non-skid footwear. Transports resident to shower or tub room.		
For a shower:			
9.	If using a shower chair, places it into position and locks its wheels. Transfers resident into shower chair.		
10.	Turns on water. Tests water temperature with thermometer. Has resident check water temperature. Adjusts if necessary. Checks water temperature frequently throughout the shower.		
For a tub bath:			
9.	Transfers resident onto chair or tub lift.		
10.	Fills the tub halfway with warm water. Tests water temperature with thermometer. Has resident check water temperature.		
Remaining steps for either procedure:			
11.	Puts on clean gloves.		
12.	Helps resident remove clothing and shoes.		
13.	Helps resident into shower or tub. Puts shower chair into shower and locks wheels.		
14.	Stays with resident during the entire procedure.		
15.	Lets resident wash as much as possible on his or her own. Helps to wash his or her face.		
16.	Helps resident shampoo hair. Rinses hair thoroughly.		

17.	Helps to wash and rinse the entire body. Moves from head to toe (clean to dirty).		
18.	Turns off water or drains tub. Covers resident with bath blanket until the tub drains.		
19.	Unlocks shower chair wheels if used. Rolls resident out of shower, or helps resident out of tub and onto a chair.		
20.	Gives resident towel(s) and helps to pat dry everywhere, including under the breasts, between skin folds, in the perineal area, and between toes.		
21.	Places soiled clothing and linens in proper containers.		
22.	Removes and discards gloves.		
23.	Washes hands.		
24.	Applies lotion and deodorant as needed. Helps resident dress and comb hair before leaving shower or tub room. Puts on non-skid footwear. Returns resident to room.		
25.	Makes resident comfortable.		
26.	Leaves call light within resident's reach.		
27.	Washes hands.		
28.	Is courteous and respectful at all times.		
29.	Reports any changes in resident to the nurse. Documents procedure using facility guidelines.		

_____   _____
Date Reviewed   Instructor Signature

_____   _____
Date Performed   Instructor Signature

Giving a back rub

		yes	no
1.	Identifies self by name. Identifies resident. Greets resident by name.		

2.	Washes hands.		
3.	Explains procedure to resident. Speaks clearly, slowly, and directly. Maintains face-to-face contact whenever possible.		
4.	Provides for resident's privacy with a curtain, screen, or door.		
5.	Adjusts bed to a safe level, usually waist high. Locks bed wheels.		
6.	Positions resident lying on his side (lateral position) or his stomach (prone position). Covers with a bath blanket. Exposes back to the top of the buttocks.		
7.	Warms lotion by putting bottle in warm water for five minutes. Runs hands under warm water. Pours lotion on hands. Rubs them together.		
8.	Places hands on each side of upper part of the buttocks. Uses full palm of hand. Makes long, smooth, upward strokes with both hands. Moves along each side of the spine, up to the shoulders. Circles hands outward. Moves back along outer edges of the back. At buttocks, makes another circle. Moves hands back up to the shoulders. Without taking hands from resident's skin, repeats this motion for three to five minutes.		
9.	Kneads with the first two fingers and thumb of each hand. Places them at base of the spine. Moves upward together along each side of the spine. Applies gentle downward pressure with fingers and thumbs. Follows same direction as with the long smooth strokes, circling at shoulders and buttocks.		

Name: _____

10.	Massages bony areas (spine, shoulder blades, hip bones). Uses circular motions of fingertips. Does not massage any pale, white, or red areas.		
11.	Finishes with long, smooth strokes.		
12.	Dries the back if it has extra lotion remaining.		
13.	Removes bath blanket. Helps resident to get dressed. Makes resident comfortable.		
14.	Returns bed to lowest position. Removes privacy measures.		
15.	Stores supplies. Places soiled clothing and linens in proper containers.		
16.	Leaves call light within resident's reach.		
17.	Washes hands.		
18.	Is courteous and respectful at all times.		
19.	Reports any changes in the resident to the nurse, including pale, white, or red areas. Documents procedure using facility guidelines.		

_____   _____
Date Reviewed   Instructor Signature

_____   _____
Date Performed   Instructor Signature

Providing oral care

		yes	no
	Maintains clean technique with placement of toothbrush throughout procedure.		
1.	Identifies self by name. Identifies resident. Greets resident by name.		
2.	Washes hands.		
3.	Explains procedure to resident. Speaks clearly, slowly, and directly. Maintains face-to-face contact whenever possible.		

4.	Provides for resident's privacy with a curtain, screen, or door.		
5.	Adjusts bed to safe working level, usually waist high. Locks bed wheels. Makes sure resident is sitting upright.		
6.	Puts on gloves.		
7.	Places towel across resident's chest.		
8.	Wets brush. Applies toothpaste.		
9.	Cleans entire mouth (including tongue and all surfaces of teeth and the gumline) using gentle strokes. First brushes inner, outer and chewing surfaces of the upper teeth, then does the same with the lower teeth. Uses short strokes. Brushes back and forth.		
10.	Holds emesis basin to the resident's chin.		
11.	Has resident rinse mouth with water and spit into emesis basin.		
12.	Wipes resident's mouth and removes towel.		
13.	Empties, rinses, and wipes emesis basin. Rinses toothbrush. Returns supplies to proper storage.		
14.	Disposes of soiled linen in the proper container.		
15.	Removes and discards gloves. Washes hands.		
16.	Makes resident comfortable.		
17.	Returns bed to lowest position. Removes privacy measures.		
18.	Leaves call light within resident's reach.		
19.	Washes hands.		
20.	Is courteous and respectful at all times.		

21.	Reports any changes in resident to the nurse. Reports any problems with teeth, mouth, tongue, or lips to nurse. This includes odor, cracking, sores, bleeding, and any discoloration. Documents procedure using facility guidelines.		

_____   _____
Date Reviewed   Instructor Signature

_____   _____
Date Performed   Instructor Signature

Flossing teeth

		yes	no
1.	Identifies self by name. Identifies resident. Greets resident by name.		
2.	Washes hands.		
3.	Explains procedure to resident. Speaks clearly, slowly, and directly. Maintains face-to-face contact whenever possible.		
4.	Provides for resident's privacy with a curtain, screen, or door.		
5.	Adjusts bed to safe working level, usually waist high. Locks bed wheels. Makes sure resident is in an upright sitting position.		
6.	Puts on gloves.		
7.	Wraps ends of floss securely around each index finger.		
8.	Starting with the back teeth, places floss between teeth. Moves it down the surface of the tooth. Uses a gentle sawing motion.		
	Continues to the gum line. At the gum line, curves the floss. Slips it gently into the space between the gum and tooth. Then goes back up, scraping that side of the tooth. Repeats on the side of the other tooth.		

9.	After every two teeth, unwinds floss from fingers. Moves floss to use a clean area. Flosses all teeth.		
10.	Offers water to rinse the mouth. Asks resident to spit it into the basin.		
11.	Offers resident a face towel when done.		
12.	Discards floss. Empties basin into the toilet. Cleans and stores basin and supplies.		
13.	Disposes of soiled linen in the proper container.		
14.	Removes and discards gloves. Washes hands.		
15.	Makes resident comfortable.		
16.	Returns bed to lowest position. Removes privacy measures.		
17.	Leaves call light within resident's reach.		
18.	Washes hands.		
19.	Is courteous and respectful at all times.		
20.	Reports any changes in resident to the nurse. Reports any problems with teeth, mouth, tongue, or lips to nurse. This includes odor, cracking, sores, bleeding, and any discoloration. Documents procedure using facility guidelines.		

_____   _____
Date Reviewed   Instructor Signature

_____   _____
Date Performed   Instructor Signature

Cleaning and storing dentures

		yes	no
	Maintains clean technique with placement of dentures and toothbrush throughout procedure.		

Name: _____

1.	Identifies self by name. Identifies resident. Greets resident by name.		
2.	Washes hands.		
3.	Explains procedure to resident. Speaks clearly, slowly, and directly. Maintains face-to-face contact whenever possible.		
4.	Provides for resident's privacy with a curtain, screen, or door.		
5.	Adjusts bed to safe working level, usually waist high. Locks bed wheels. Makes sure resident is in an upright sitting position.		
6.	Puts on gloves.		
7.	Lines sink/basin with a towel(s) and partially fills sink with water.		
8.	If removing dentures, removes lower denture first. Grasps lower denture with a gauze square and removes it. Firmly grasps upper denture with a gauze square. Gives a slight downward pull to break the suction. Turns it at an angle to take it out of the mouth.		
9.	Rinses dentures in tepid/lukewarm running water before brushing them.		
10.	Applies toothpaste or cleanser to toothbrush.		
11.	Brushes dentures on all surfaces.		
12.	Rinses all surfaces of dentures under tepid/lukewarm running water.		
13.	Offers water to rinse the resident's mouth. Asks resident to spit it into the emesis basin.		
14.	Rinses denture cup if placing clean dentures inside it.		
15.	Places dentures in clean denture cup with special solution or lukewarm water and cover. Makes sure cup is labeled with resident's name. Returns denture cup to storage.		

16.	If replacing dentures in resident's mouth, makes sure resident is still sitting upright. Applies denture cream or adhesive to the dentures, if needed. When the resident's mouth is open, places upper denture into the mouth by turning it at an angle. Straightens it. Presses it onto the upper gum line firmly and evenly. Inserts lower denture onto the gum line of the lower jaw. Presses firmly.		
17.	Cleans, dries, and returns equipment to proper storage.		
18.	Disposes of soiled linen in the proper container and drains sink.		
19.	Removes and discards gloves. Washes hands.		
20.	Makes resident comfortable.		
21.	Returns bed to lowest position. Removes privacy measures.		
22.	Leaves call light within resident's reach.		
23.	Washes hands.		
24.	Is courteous and respectful at all times.		
25.	Reports any changes in resident or the appearance of dentures to the nurse. Documents procedure using facility guidelines.		

_____   _____
Date Reviewed   Instructor Signature

_____   _____
Date Performed   Instructor Signature

Providing oral care for the unconscious resident

		yes	no
1.	Identifies self by name. Identifies resident. Greets resident by name.		
2.	Washes hands.		

3.	Explains procedure to resident. Speaks clearly, slowly, and directly. Maintains face-to-face contact whenever possible.		
4.	Provides for resident's privacy with a curtain, screen, or door.		
5.	Adjusts bed to a safe level, usually waist high. Locks bed wheels.		
6.	Puts on gloves.		
7.	Turns resident on his side or turns head to the side. Places a towel under his cheek and chin. Places an emesis basin next to the cheek and chin for excess fluid.		
8.	Holds mouth open with tongue depressor. Does not use fingers to open the mouth or keep it open.		
9.	Dips swab in cleaning solution. Squeezes excess solution to prevent aspiration. Wipes inner, outer, and chewing surfaces of the upper and lower teeth, gums, tongue, and inside surfaces of mouth. Changes swab often. Repeats until the mouth is clean.		
10.	Rinses with clean swab dipped in water. Squeezes swab first to remove excess water.		
11.	Removes towel and basin. Pats lips or face dry. Applies lip lubricant.		
12.	Cleans and returns supplies to proper storage.		
13.	Disposes of soiled linen in the proper container.		
14.	Removes and discards gloves. Washes hands.		
15.	Makes resident comfortable.		
16.	Returns bed to lowest position. Removes privacy measures.		
17.	Leaves call light within resident's reach.		

18.	Washes hands.		
19.	Is courteous and respectful at all times.		
20.	Reports any changes in resident to the nurse. Reports any problems with teeth, mouth, tongue, or lips to nurse. This includes odor, cracking, sores, bleeding, and any discoloration. Documents procedure using facility guidelines.		

_____   _____
Date Reviewed   Instructor Signature

_____   _____
Date Performed   Instructor Signature

Shaving a resident			
		yes	no
1.	Identifies self by name. Identifies resident. Greets resident by name.		
2.	Washes hands.		
3.	Explains procedure to resident. Speaks clearly, slowly, and directly. Maintains face-to-face contact whenever possible.		
4.	Provides for resident's privacy with a curtain, screen, or door.		
5.	Adjusts bed to a safe level, usually waist high. Locks bed wheels.		
6.	Raises head of bed so resident is sitting up. Places towel across the resident's chest, under his chin.		
7.	Puts on gloves.		
	Shaving using a safety or disposable razor:		
8.	Softens beard with a warm, wet washcloth on the face for a few minutes before shaving. Lathers the face with shaving cream or soap and warm water.		

9.	Holds skin taut. Shaves in direction of the hair growth. Shaves beard in short, downward, and even strokes on face and upward strokes on neck. Rinses the blade often in warm water to keep it clean and wet.		
10.	When finished, washes, rinses, and dries resident's face with a warm, wet washcloth. Offers mirror to resident.		
	Shaving using an electric razor:		
8.	Uses a small brush to clean razor, if necessary. Does not use an electric razor near any water source, when oxygen is in use, or if resident has a pacemaker.		
9.	Turns on the razor and holds skin taut. Shaves with smooth, even movements. Shaves beard with back and forth motion in direction of beard growth with foil shaver. Shaves beard in circular motion with three-head shaver. Shaves the chin and under the chin.		
10.	Offers mirror to resident.		
	Final steps:		
11.	Applies after-shave lotion as resident wishes.		
12.	Removes towel and places towel and washcloth in proper container.		
13.	Cleans equipment and stores it. **For safety razor**: rinses razor and stores it. **For disposable razor**: disposes of it in a sharps container. Does not recap razor. **For electric razor**: cleans head of razor. Removes whiskers from razor. Recaps shaving head. Returns razor to case.		
14.	Removes and discards gloves. Washes hands.		
15.	Makes sure that there are no loose hairs. Makes resident comfortable.		

16.	Returns bed to lowest position. Removes privacy measures.		
17.	Leaves call light within resident's reach.		
18.	Washes hands.		
19.	Is courteous and respectful at all times.		
20.	Reports any changes in resident to the nurse. Documents procedure using facility guidelines.		

_____   _____
Date Reviewed   Instructor Signature

_____   _____
Date Performed   Instructor Signature

Providing fingernail care

		yes	no
1.	Identifies self by name. Identifies resident. Greets resident by name.		
2.	Washes hands.		
3.	Explains procedure to resident. Speaks clearly, slowly, and directly. Maintains face-to-face contact whenever possible.		
4.	Provides for resident's privacy with a curtain, screen, or door.		
5.	If the resident is in bed, adjusts bed to safe working level, usually waist high. Locks bed wheels.		
6.	Fills basin halfway with warm water. Tests water temperature with thermometer or wrist. Ensures it is safe. Has resident check water temperature. Adjusts if necessary. Places basin at a comfortable level for resident.		
7.	Puts on gloves.		
8.	Soaks resident's nails in the basin of water. Soaks all 10 fingertips for at least five minutes.		

9.	Removes hands from basin. Washes hands with soapy washcloth. Rinses. Pats hands dry with towel, including between fingers. Removes hand basin.		
10.	Places resident's hands on the towel. Gently cleans under each fingernail with orangewood stick.		
11.	Wipes orangewood stick on towel after each nail. Washes resident's hands again. Dries them thoroughly, especially between fingers.		
12.	Shapes nails with file or emery board. Files in a curve. Finishes with nails smooth and free of rough edges.		
13.	Empties, rinses, and wipes basin. Places basin in proper area for cleaning or cleans and stores it according to policy.		
14.	Disposes of soiled linen in the proper container.		
15.	Removes and discards gloves. Washes hands.		
16.	Makes resident comfortable.		
17.	Returns bed to lowest position. Removes privacy measures.		
18.	Leaves call light within resident's reach.		
19.	Washes hands.		
20.	Is courteous and respectful at all times.		
21.	Reports any changes in resident to the nurse. Documents procedure using facility guidelines.		

_____   _____
Date Reviewed   Instructor Signature

_____   _____
Date Performed   Instructor Signature

Combing or brushing hair

		yes	no
	Uses hair care products that the resident prefers for his or her type of hair.		
1.	Identifies self by name. Identifies resident. Greets resident by name.		
2.	Washes hands.		
3.	Explains procedure to resident. Speaks clearly, slowly, and directly. Maintains face-to-face contact whenever possible.		
4.	Provides for resident's privacy with a curtain, screen, or door.		
5.	If the resident is in bed, adjusts bed to safe working level, usually waist high. Locks bed wheels.		
6.	Raises head of bed so resident is sitting up. Places towel under head or around shoulders.		
7.	Removes any hair pins, hair ties, and clips.		
8.	Removes tangles first by dividing hair into small sections. Combs out from ends to roots of hair.		
9.	After tangles are removed, brushes two-inch sections of hair at a time. Brushes from ends to roots.		
10.	Neatly styles hair as resident prefers. Avoids childish hairstyles. Offers mirror to resident.		
11.	Makes resident comfortable.		
12.	Returns bed to lowest position. Removes privacy measures.		
13.	Returns supplies to proper storage. Cleans hair from brush/comb. Cleans comb and brush.		
14.	Disposes of soiled linen in the proper container.		
15.	Leaves call light within resident's reach.		
16.	Washes hands.		

| 17. | Is courteous and respectful at all times. | | |
| 18. | Reports any changes in resident to the nurse. Documents procedure using facility guidelines. | | |

_____ _____
Date Reviewed   Instructor Signature

_____ _____
Date Performed   Instructor Signature

Dressing a resident			
		yes	no
	When putting on all items, moves resident's body gently and naturally. Avoids force and over-extension of limbs and joints.		
1.	Identifies self by name. Identifies resident. Greets resident by name.		
2.	Washes hands.		
3.	Explains procedure to resident. Speaks clearly, slowly, and directly. Maintains face-to-face contact whenever possible.		
4.	Provides for resident's privacy with a curtain, screen, or door.		
5.	Asks resident what she would like to wear. Dresses her in outfit of choice.		
6.	Removes resident's gown. Does not completely expose resident. Takes clothes off stronger side first when undressing. Then removes from weaker side.		
7.	Gathers up sleeve to ease pulling over affected arm. Inserts hand through sleeve and grasps resident's hand to support arm while dressing. Assists resident to put the affected/weaker arm through the sleeve of the shirt, sweater, or slip before placing garment on the unaffected/stronger arm.		

8.	Helps resident to put on skirt, pants, or dress. Puts affected/weak leg through skirt or pants first. Raises buttocks or turns resident from side to side to draw pants over the buttocks up to waist.		
9.	Places bed at the lowest position. Locks bed wheels.		
10.	Has resident sit down. Pulls up socks until they are both smooth and without wrinkles. Puts on non-skid footwear. Fastens securely.		
11.	Finishes with resident dressed appropriately. Makes sure clothing is right-side out and zippers/buttons are fastened.		
12.	Makes resident comfortable. Removes privacy measures.		
13.	Places gown in soiled linen container.		
14.	Leaves call light within resident's reach.		
15.	Washes hands.		
16.	Is courteous and respectful at all times.		
17.	Reports any changes in resident to the nurse. Documents procedure using facility guidelines.		

_____ _____
Date Reviewed   Instructor Signature

_____ _____
Date Performed   Instructor Signature

13
Vital Signs

Measuring and recording oral temperature			
		yes	no
	Does not take an oral temperature on a resident who has smoked, eaten or drunk fluids, chewed gum, or exercised within the last 10–20 minutes.		

1.	Identifies self by name. Identifies resident. Greets resident by name.		
2.	Washes hands.		
3.	Explains procedure to resident. Speaks clearly, slowly, and directly. Maintains face-to-face contact whenever possible.		
4.	Provides for resident's privacy with a curtain, screen, or door.		
5.	Puts on gloves.		
6.	**Mercury-free thermometer**: Holds thermometer by stem. Before inserting thermometer in resident's mouth, shakes thermometer down to below the lowest number (at least below 96°F or 35°C).		
	Digital thermometer: Puts on disposable sheath. Turns on thermometer. Waits until "ready" sign appears.		
	Electronic thermometer: Removes probe from base unit. Puts on probe cover.		
7.	**Mercury-free thermometer**: Puts on disposable sheath, if applicable. Gently inserts bulb end of thermometer into resident's mouth. Places it under tongue and to one side.		
	Digital thermometer: Inserts end of digital thermometer into resident's mouth. Places under tongue and to one side.		
	Electronic thermometer: Inserts the covered probe into resident's mouth. Places under tongue and to one side.		
8.	**Mercury-free thermometer**: Tells resident to hold thermometer in mouth with lips closed. Assists as necessary. Asks resident not to bite down or to talk. Leaves thermometer in place for at least three minutes.		

	Digital thermometer: Leaves in place until thermometer blinks or beeps.		
	Electronic thermometer: Leaves in place until a tone is heard or a flashing or steady light is seen.		
9.	**Mercury-free thermometer**: Removes thermometer. Wipes with tissue from stem to bulb or remove sheath. Disposes of tissue or sheath. Holds thermometer at eye level. Rotates until line appears, rolling the thermometer between thumb and forefinger. Reads temperature. Remembers temperature reading.		
	Digital thermometer: Removes thermometer. Reads temperature on display screen. Remembers temperature reading.		
	Electronic thermometer: Reads temperature on the display screen. Remembers temperature reading. Removes probe.		
10.	**Mercury-free thermometer**: Cleans thermometer according to policy. Returns it to plastic case or container.		
	Digital thermometer: Using a tissue, removes and discards sheath. Cleans thermometer according to policy. Replaces thermometer in case.		
	Electronic thermometer: Presses eject button to discard the cover. Returns probe to the holder.		
11.	Removes and discards gloves. Washes hands.		
12.	Makes resident comfortable. Removes privacy measures.		
13.	Leaves call light within resident's reach.		
14.	Washes hands.		
15.	Is courteous and respectful at all times.		

16.	Reports any changes in resident to the nurse. Documents procedure using facility guidelines. Records resident's name, temperature, date, time and method used (oral).		

_____	_____
Date Reviewed	Instructor Signature

_____	_____
Date Performed	Instructor Signature

Measuring and recording rectal temperature

		yes	no
1.	Identifies self by name. Identifies resident. Greets resident by name.		
2.	Washes hands.		
3.	Explains procedure to resident. Speaks clearly, slowly, and directly. Maintains face-to-face contact whenever possible.		
4.	Provides for resident's privacy with a curtain, screen, or door.		
5.	Adjusts bed to a safe level, usually waist high. Locks bed wheels.		
6.	Helps resident to left-lying (Sims') position.		
7.	Folds back linens to expose only rectal area.		
8.	Puts on gloves.		
9.	*Mercury-free glass thermometer*: Holds thermometer by stem. Shakes thermometer down to below the lowest number. Puts on disposable sheath.		
	Digital thermometer: Puts on disposable sheath. Turns on thermometer. Waits until "ready" sign appears.		
	Electronic thermometer: Removes probe from base unit. Puts on probe cover.		

10.	Applies a small amount of lubricant to tip of bulb or probe cover (or applies pre-lubricated cover).		
11.	Separates the buttocks. Gently inserts thermometer one-half to one inch into rectum. Stops if resistance is met. Does not force thermometer into rectum.		
12.	Replaces sheet over buttocks while holding on to thermometer. Holds onto thermometer at all times.		
13.	*Mercury-free glass thermometer*: Holds thermometer in place for at least three minutes.		
	Digital thermometer: Holds thermometer in place until thermometer blinks or beeps.		
	Electronic thermometer: Leaves in place until a tone is heard or a flashing or steady light is seen.		
14.	Gently removes thermometer. Wipes with tissue from stem to bulb or removes sheath or cover. Disposes of tissue or sheath.		
15.	Reads thermometer at eye level. Remembers temperature reading.		
16.	*Mercury-free glass thermometer*: Cleans thermometer according to policy. Returns it to plastic case or container.		
	Digital thermometer: Cleans thermometer according to policy. Replaces thermometer in case.		
	Electronic thermometer: Presses eject button to discard the cover. Returns probe to holder.		
17.	Removes and discards gloves.		
18.	Washes hands.		
19.	Makes resident comfortable.		
20.	Returns bed to lowest position. Removes privacy measures.		

21.	Leaves call light within resident's reach.		
22.	Washes hands.		
23.	Is courteous and respectful at all times.		
24.	Reports any changes in resident to the nurse. Documents procedure using facility guidelines. Records resident's name, temperature, date, time and method used (rectal).		

_____   _____
Date Reviewed   Instructor Signature

_____   _____
Date Performed   Instructor Signature

Measuring and recording tympanic temperature

		yes	no
1.	Identifies self by name. Identifies resident. Greets resident by name.		
2.	Washes hands.		
3.	Explains procedure to resident. Speaks clearly, slowly, and directly. Maintains face-to-face contact whenever possible.		
4.	Provides for resident's privacy with a curtain, screen, or door.		
5.	Puts on gloves.		
6.	Puts a disposable sheath over earpiece of the thermometer.		
7.	Positions resident's head so that the ear is in front of self. Straightens ear canal by gently pulling up and back on the outside edge of the ear. Inserts covered probe into the ear canal. Presses button.		
8.	Holds thermometer in place until thermometer blinks or beeps.		
9.	Reads temperature. Remembers temperature reading.		

10.	Disposes of sheath. Returns thermometer to storage or to the battery charger if thermometer is rechargeable.		
11.	Removes and discards gloves. Washes hands.		
12.	Makes resident comfortable. Removes privacy measures.		
13.	Leaves call light within resident's reach.		
14.	Washes hands.		
15.	Is courteous and respectful at all times.		
16.	Reports any changes in resident to the nurse. Documents procedure using facility guidelines. Records resident's name, temperature, date, time, and method used (tympanic).		

_____   _____
Date Reviewed   Instructor Signature

_____   _____
Date Performed   Instructor Signature

Measuring and recording axillary temperature

		yes	no
1.	Identifies self by name. Identifies resident. Greets resident by name.		
2.	Washes hands.		
3.	Explains procedure to resident. Speaks clearly, slowly, and directly. Maintains face-to-face contact whenever possible.		
4.	Provides for resident's privacy with a curtain, screen, or door.		
5.	Adjusts bed to a safe level, usually waist high. Locks bed wheels.		
6.	Puts on gloves.		
7.	Removes resident's arm from sleeve of gown. Wipes axillary area with tissues.		

8.	**Mercury-free glass thermometer**: Holds thermometer by stem. Shakes thermometer down to below the lowest number. Puts on disposable sheath, if applicable.		
	Digital thermometer: Puts on disposable sheath. Turns on thermometer. Waits until "ready" sign appears.		
	Electronic thermometer: Removes probe from base unit. Puts on probe cover.		
9.	Positions thermometer (bulb end for mercury-free) in center of the armpit. Folds resident's arm over chest.		
10.	**Mercury-free glass thermometer**: Holds thermometer in place, with the arm close against the side, for eight to ten minutes.		
	Digital thermometer: Holds thermometer in place until thermometer blinks or beeps.		
	Electronic thermometer: Leaves in place until a tone is heard or a flashing or steady light is seen.		
11.	**Mercury-free glass thermometer**: Removes thermometer. Wipes with tissue from stem to bulb or remove sheath. Disposes of tissue or sheath. Reads temperature. Remembers temperature reading.		
	Digital thermometer: Removes thermometer. Reads temperature on display screen. Remembers temperature reading.		
	Electronic thermometer: Reads temperature on the display screen. Remembers temperature reading. Removes probe.		
12.	**Mercury-free thermometer**: Cleans thermometer according to policy. Returns it to plastic case or container.		

	Digital thermometer: Using a tissue, removes and disposes of sheath. Cleans thermometer according to policy. Replaces thermometer in case.		
	Electronic thermometer: Presses eject button to discard the cover. Returns probe to the holder.		
13.	Removes and discards gloves. Washes hands.		
14.	Puts resident's arm back into sleeve of gown. Makes resident comfortable.		
15.	Returns bed to lowest position. Removes privacy measures.		
16.	Leaves call light within resident's reach.		
17.	Washes hands.		
18.	Is courteous and respectful at all times.		
19.	Reports any changes in resident to the nurse. Documents procedure using facility guidelines. Records resident's name, temperature, date, time and method used (axillary).		

_____   _____
Date Reviewed   Instructor Signature

_____   _____
Date Performed   Instructor Signature

Measuring and recording radial pulse and counting and recording respirations

		yes	no
1.	Identifies self by name. Identifies resident. Greets resident by name.		
2.	Washes hands.		
3.	Explains procedure to resident. Speaks clearly, slowly, and directly. Maintains face-to-face contact whenever possible.		
4.	Provides for resident's privacy with a curtain, screen, or door.		

5.	Places fingertips of index finger and middle finger on the thumb side of resident's wrist to locate radial pulse. Does not use thumb.		
6.	Counts beats for one full minute.		
7.	Keeps fingertips on resident's wrist. Counts respirations for one full minute. Observes for pattern and character of resident's breathing.		
8.	Removes privacy measures. Makes resident comfortable.		
9.	Leaves call light within resident's reach.		
10.	Washes hands.		
11.	Is courteous and respectful at all times.		
12.	Reports any changes in resident to the nurse. Documents procedure using facility guidelines. Records pulse rate, date, time and method used (radial). Records respiratory rate and pattern or character of breathing.		

_____   _____
Date Reviewed   Instructor Signature

_____   _____
Date Performed   Instructor Signature

5.	Before using stethoscope, wipes diaphragm and earpieces with alcohol wipes.		
6.	Fits earpieces of the stethoscope snugly in ears. Places flat metal diaphragm on the left side of the chest, just below the nipple. Listens for the heartbeat.		
7.	Uses second hand of watch. Counts beats for one full minute. Leaves stethoscope in place to count respirations.		
8.	Cleans earpieces and diaphragm of stethoscope with alcohol wipes. Stores stethoscope.		
9.	Makes resident comfortable. Removes privacy measures.		
10.	Leaves call light within resident's reach.		
11.	Washes hands.		
12.	Is courteous and respectful at all times.		
13.	Reports any changes in resident to the nurse. Documents procedure using facility guidelines. Records pulse rate, date, time, and method used (apical). Notes any differences in rhythm.		

_____   _____
Date Reviewed   Instructor Signature

_____   _____
Date Performed   Instructor Signature

Measuring and recording apical pulse

		yes	no
1.	Identifies self by name. Identifies resident. Greets resident by name.		
2.	Washes hands.		
3.	Explains procedure to resident. Speaks clearly, slowly, and directly. Maintains face-to-face contact whenever possible.		
4.	Provides for resident's privacy with a curtain, screen, or door.		

Measuring and recording apical-radial pulse

		yes	no
	Finds co-worker to assist.		
1.	Identifies self by name. Identifies resident. Greets resident by name.		
2.	Washes hands.		
3.	Explains procedure to resident. Speaks clearly, slowly, and directly. Maintains face-to-face contact whenever possible.		

4.	Provides for resident's privacy with a curtain, screen, or door.		
5.	Before using stethoscope, wipes diaphragm and earpieces with alcohol wipes.		
6.	Fits earpieces of stethoscope snugly in ears. Places flat metal diaphragm on the left side of the chest, just below the nipple. Listens for the heartbeat.		
7.	Co-worker places her fingertips on the thumb side of resident's wrist to locate the radial pulse.		
8.	After both pulses have been located, looks at the second hand of watch. When the second hand reaches the "12" or "6," says, "Start," and both people count beats for one full minute. Says, "Stop" after one minute.		
9.	Cleans earpieces and diaphragm of stethoscope with alcohol wipes. Stores stethoscope.		
10.	Makes resident comfortable. Removes privacy measures.		
11.	Leaves call light within resident's reach.		
12.	Washes hands.		
13.	Is courteous and respectful at all times.		
14.	Reports any changes in resident to the nurse. Documents procedure using facility guidelines. Records both pulse rates, date, time, and method used (apical-radial). Records pulse deficit if the pulse rates are not the same. Notes any differences in rhythm.		

_____   _____
Date Reviewed   Instructor Signature

_____   _____
Date Performed   Instructor Signature

Measuring and recording blood pressure (one-step method)

		yes	no
1.	Identifies self by name. Identifies resident. Greets resident by name.		
2.	Washes hands.		
3.	Explains procedure to resident. Speaks clearly, slowly, and directly. Maintains face-to-face contact whenever possible.		
4.	Provides for resident's privacy with a curtain, screen, or door.		
5.	Asks resident to roll up his or her sleeve, approximately five inches above the elbow. Does not measure blood pressure over clothing.		
6.	Positions resident's arm with palm up, with arm level with the heart.		
7.	With the valve open, squeezes the cuff. Makes sure it is completely deflated.		
8.	Places blood pressure cuff snugly on resident's upper arm. Makes sure center of the cuff with sensor/arrow is placed over the brachial artery (1-1½ inches above the elbow toward inside of elbow).		
9.	Before using the stethoscope, wipes diaphragm and earpieces with alcohol wipes.		
10.	Locates brachial pulse with fingertips.		
11.	Places diaphragm of the stethoscope over brachial artery.		
12.	Places earpieces of the stethoscope in ears.		
13.	Closes the valve (clockwise) until it stops. Does not over-tighten it.		

14.	Inflates cuff to 30 mm Hg above the point at which the pulse is last heard or felt.		
15.	Opens valve slightly with thumb and index finger. Deflates cuff slowly.		
16.	Watches gauge. Listens for sound of pulse.		
17.	Remembers reading at which the first clear pulse sound is heard. This is the systolic pressure.		
18.	Continues listening for a change or muffling of pulse sound. The point of a change or the point the sound disappears is the diastolic pressure. Remembers this reading.		
19.	Opens the valve. Deflates cuff completely. Removes cuff.		
20.	Wipes diaphragm and earpieces of the stethoscope with alcohol. Stores equipment.		
21.	Makes resident comfortable. Removes privacy measures.		
22.	Leaves call light within resident's reach.		
23.	Washes hands.		
24.	Is courteous and respectful at all times.		
25.	Reports any changes in resident to the nurse. Documents procedure using facility guidelines. Records both the systolic and diastolic pressures. Writes the numbers like a fraction, with the systolic reading on top and the diastolic reading on the bottom (for example: 120/80). Notes which arm was used. Writes "RA" for right arm and "LA" for left arm.		

_____   _____
Date Reviewed   Instructor Signature

_____   _____
Date Performed   Instructor Signature

Measuring and recording blood pressure (two-step method)

		yes	no
1.	Identifies self by name. Identifies resident. Greets resident by name.		
2.	Washes hands.		
3.	Explains procedure to resident. Speaks clearly, slowly, and directly. Maintains face-to-face contact whenever possible.		
4.	Provides for resident's privacy with a curtain, screen, or door.		
5.	Asks resident to roll up his or her sleeve, approximately five inches above the elbow. Does not measure blood pressure over clothing.		
6.	Positions resident's arm with palm up, with arm level with the heart.		
7.	With the valve open, squeezes the cuff. Makes sure it is completely deflated.		
8.	Places blood pressure cuff snugly on resident's upper arm. Makes sure center of the cuff with sensor/arrow is placed over the brachial artery (1-1½ inches above the elbow toward inside of elbow).		
9.	Locates radial (wrist) pulse with fingertips.		
10.	Closes valve (clockwise) until it stops. Inflates cuff slowly, watching gauge.		
11.	Stops inflating when pulse is no longer felt. Notes reading. The number is an estimate of the systolic pressure.		
12.	Opens valve. Deflates cuff completely.		
13.	Writes down estimated systolic reading.		

14.	Before using the stethoscope, wipes diaphragm and earpieces of stethoscope with alcohol wipes.		
15.	Locates brachial pulse with fingertips.		
16.	Places diaphragm of the stethoscope over brachial artery.		
17.	Places earpieces of the stethoscope in ears.		
18.	Closes valve (clockwise) until it stops. Does not over-tighten it.		
19.	Inflates cuff to 30 mm Hg above estimated systolic pressure.		
20.	Opens valve slightly with thumb and index finger. Deflates cuff slowly.		
21.	Watches gauge. Listens for sound of pulse.		
22.	Remembers reading at which first clear pulse sound is heard. This is the systolic pressure.		
23.	Continues listening for a change or muffling of pulse sound. The point of a change or the point the sound disappears is the diastolic pressure. Remembers this reading.		
24.	Opens valve. Deflates cuff completely. Removes cuff.		
25.	Wipes diaphragm and earpieces of the stethoscope with alcohol. Stores equipment.		
26.	Makes resident comfortable. Removes privacy measures.		
27.	Leaves call light within resident's reach.		
28.	Washes hands.		
29.	Is courteous and respectful at all times.		

30.	Reports any changes in resident to the nurse. Documents procedure using facility guidelines. Records both the systolic and diastolic pressures. Writes the numbers like a fraction, with the systolic reading on top and the diastolic reading on the bottom (for example: 120/80). Notes which arm was used. Writes "RA" for right arm and "LA" for left arm.		

_____ _____
Date Reviewed   Instructor Signature

_____ _____
Date Performed   Instructor Signature

14
Nutrition and Fluid Balance

Feeding a resident who cannot feed self		yes	no
1.	Identifies self by name. Identifies resident. Greets resident by name.		
2.	Washes hands.		
3.	Explains procedure to resident. Speaks clearly, slowly, and directly. Maintains face-to-face contact whenever possible.		
4.	Provides for resident's privacy with a curtain, screen, or door.		
5.	Picks up diet card. Asks resident to state his or her name. Verifies that resident has received the right tray.		
6.	Raises head of the bed. Makes sure resident is in an upright sitting position (at a 90-degree angle).		
7.	Adjusts bed height so that caregiver is at resident's eye level. Locks bed wheels.		
8.	Places meal tray where it can be easily seen by the resident, such as on the overbed table.		

9.	Helps resident to clean hands with hand wipes if resident cannot do it on her own.		
10.	Helps resident to put on clothing protector, if desired.		
11.	Sits facing resident. Sits at resident's eye level. Sits on the stronger side if resident has one-sided weakness.		
12.	Tells resident what foods are on tray. Offers a drink of beverage and asks what resident would like to eat first.		
13.	Offers food in bite-sized pieces, telling the resident the content of each bite of food offered. Alternates types of food, allowing for resident's preferences. Does not feed all of one type before offering another type. Reports any swallowing problems to the nurse immediately. If resident has one-sided weakness, directs food to the stronger side.		
14.	Offers sips of beverage to resident throughout the meal.		
15.	Makes sure resident's mouth is empty before next bite or sip.		
16.	Talks with resident during the meal.		
17.	Uses washcloths or wipes to wipe food from resident's mouth and hands as needed during the meal. Wipes again at the end of the meal.		
18.	Removes clothing protector if used. Disposes of in proper container.		
19.	Removes food tray. Checks for eyeglasses, dentures, hearing aids, or any personal items before removing tray. Places tray in proper area to be picked up.		

20.	Makes resident comfortable. Makes sure the bed is free from crumbs.		
21.	Returns bed to lowest position. Removes privacy measures.		
22.	Leaves call light within resident's reach.		
23.	Washes hands.		
24.	Is courteous and respectful at all times.		
25.	Reports any changes in resident to the nurse. Documents procedure using facility guidelines. Records intake of solid food and fluids properly.		

_____   _____
Date Reviewed   Instructor Signature

_____   _____
Date Performed   Instructor Signature

Measuring and recording intake and output

		yes	no
	Measures intake first.		
1.	Identifies self by name. Identifies resident. Greets resident by name.		
2.	Washes hands.		
3.	Explains procedure to resident. Speaks clearly, slowly, and directly. Maintains face-to-face contact whenever possible.		
4.	Provides for resident's privacy with a curtain, screen, or door.		
5.	Notes amount of fluid resident is served on paper.		
6.	When the resident has finished a meal or snack, measures any leftover fluids. Notes this amount on paper.		
7.	Subtracts leftover amount from the amount served. Converts to milliliters (mL) by multiplying by 30.		

8.	Records amount of fluid consumed (in mL) in input column on I&O sheet. Records time and what fluid was consumed.		
9.	Washes hands.		
	Measures output.		
1.	Washes hands.		
2.	Puts on gloves before handling bedpan/urinal.		
3.	Pours contents of the bedpan or urinal into measuring container. Does not spill or splash any of the urine.		
4.	Places container on flat surface. Measures amount of urine at eye level. Keeps container level.		
5.	After measuring urine, empties contents of measuring container into toilet. Does not splash. Flushes toilet.		
6.	Places container and bedpan in area for cleaning or cleans and stores according to policy.		
7.	Removes and discards gloves.		
8.	Washes hands before recording output.		
9.	Records contents of container in output column on sheet. Reports any changes to the nurse.		

_____   _____
Date Reviewed   Instructor Signature

_____   _____
Date Performed   Instructor Signature

15
The Gastrointestinal System

Assisting a resident with use of a bedpan			
		yes	no
1.	Identifies self by name. Identifies resident. Greets resident by name.		
2.	Washes hands.		

3.	Explains procedure to resident. Speaks clearly, slowly, and directly. Maintains face-to-face contact whenever possible.		
4.	Provides for resident's privacy with a curtain, screen, or door.		
5.	Adjusts bed to safe level, usually waist high. Before placing bedpan, lowers head of bed. Locks bed wheels.		
6.	Puts on gloves.		
7.	Covers resident with a bath blanket. Asks him to hold it while pulling down the top covers underneath. Does not expose more of resident than is needed.		
8.	Places bed protector under resident's buttocks and hips.		
9.	Asks resident to remove undergarments or helps him do so.		
10.	Places bedpan near his hips in correct position. **Standard bedpan** should be positioned with the wider end aligned with resident's buttocks. **Fracture pan** should be positioned with handle toward foot of bed.		
11.	If resident is able, asks him to raise hips by pushing with feet and hands at the count of three. Slides bedpan under his hips.		
	If a resident cannot help in any way, keeps bed flat and rolls resident away from self. Slips bedpan under the hips and rolls him back onto bedpan. Keeps bedpan centered underneath.		
12.	Removes and discards gloves. Washes hands.		
13.	Raises head of the bed until resident is in a sitting position. Props resident into a semi-sitting position using pillows.		

14.	Places toilet tissue and wash-cloths or wipes within resident's reach. Asks resident to clean his hands with a hand wipe when finished, if he is able.		
15.	Leaves call light within resident's reach. Washes hands. Asks resident to signal when finished. Leaves room.		
16.	When called by the resident, returns and washes hands. Puts on clean gloves.		
17.	Lowers head of the bed. Makes sure resident is still covered. Does not overexpose resident.		
18.	Removes bedpan carefully. Covers bedpan. Removes bed protector.		
19.	Gives perineal care if help is needed. Wipes from front to back. Dries perineal area with a towel. Helps resident put on undergarment. Places towel in a hamper or bag, and discards disposable supplies.		
20.	Takes bedpan to the bathroom. Notes color, odor, amount, and consistency of contents. Empties contents into toilet unless the nurse needs to check the contents. Does not discard it if anything unusual about the stool or urine is noted.		
21.	Flushes toilet. Places bedpan in area for cleaning or cleans and stores it according to policy.		
22.	Removes and discards gloves. Washes hands.		
23.	Makes resident comfortable.		
24.	Returns bed to lowest position. Removes privacy measures.		
25.	Leaves call light within resident's reach.		
26.	Washes hands.		
27.	Is courteous and respectful at all times.		

28.	Reports any changes in resident to the nurse. Documents procedure using facility guidelines.		

_____   _____
Date Reviewed   Instructor Signature

_____   _____
Date Performed   Instructor Signature

Assisting a male resident with a urinal

		yes	no
1.	Identifies self by name. Identifies resident. Greets resident by name.		
2.	Washes hands.		
3.	Explains procedure to resident. Speaks clearly, slowly, and directly. Maintains face-to-face contact whenever possible.		
4.	Provides for resident's privacy with a curtain, screen, or door.		
5.	Adjusts bed to a safe level, usually waist high. Locks bed wheels.		
6.	Puts on gloves.		
7.	Places bed protector under the resident's buttocks and hips.		
8.	Hands urinal to the resident. If the resident cannot do so himself, places urinal between his legs and positions penis inside the urinal. Replaces bed covers.		
9.	Removes and discards gloves. Washes hands.		
10.	Places wipes within resident's reach. Asks resident to clean his hands with a hand wipe when finished, if he is able. Leaves call light within reach. Washes hands. Asks resident to signal when done. Leaves room.		
11.	When called by the resident, returns and washes hands. Puts on clean gloves.		

Name: _____

12.	Removes urinal. Removes bed protector. Discards disposable supplies.		
13.	Takes urinal to the bathroom. Notes color, odor, amount, and qualities of contents before flushing. Empties contents into toilet unless the nurse needs to check the contents.		
14.	Flushes toilet. Places urinal in proper area for cleaning or cleans and stores it according to policy.		
15.	Removes and discards gloves. Washes hands.		
16.	Returns bed to lowest position. Removes privacy measures.		
17.	Makes resident comfortable.		
18.	Leaves call light within resident's reach.		
19.	Washes hands.		
20.	Is courteous and respectful at all times.		
21.	Reports any changes in resident to the nurse. Documents procedure using facility guidelines.		

_____   _____
Date Reviewed   Instructor Signature

_____   _____
Date Performed   Instructor Signature

Helping a resident use a portable commode

		yes	no
1.	Identifies self by name. Identifies resident. Greets resident by name.		
2.	Washes hands.		
3.	Explains procedure to resident. Speaks clearly, slowly, and directly. Maintains face-to-face contact whenever possible.		
4.	Provides for resident's privacy with a curtain, screen, or door.		

5.	Locks commode wheels. Adjusts bed to lowest position. Locks bed wheels.		
6.	Puts on gloves.		
7.	Helps resident out of bed and to portable commode. Makes sure resident is wearing non-skid shoes and that the laces are tied.		
8.	If needed, helps resident remove clothing and sit comfortably on toilet seat. Places toilet tissue and washcloths or wipes within resident's reach. Asks resident to clean his hands with a hand wipe when finished, if he is able.		
9.	Places blanket over resident's legs. Leaves call light within resident's reach. Removes and discards gloves. Washes hands. Asks resident to signal when finished. Leaves room.		
10.	When called by the resident, returns and washes hands. Puts on clean gloves.		
11.	Gives perineal care if help is needed. Wipes from front to back. Dries perineal area with a towel. Helps resident put on undergarment. Places towel in a hamper or bag. Discards disposable supplies.		
12.	Removes and discards gloves. Washes hands.		
13.	Helps resident back to bed. Leaves bed in lowest position. Removes privacy measures.		
14.	Makes resident comfortable.		
15.	Puts on clean gloves.		
16.	Removes waste basin. Notes color, odor, amount, and consistency of contents. Empties contents into toilet unless nurse needs to check the contents.		

17.	Flushes toilet. Places container in proper area for cleaning or cleans it according to facility policy.		
18.	Removes and discards gloves. Washes hands.		
19.	Leaves call light within resident's reach.		
20.	Washes hands.		
21.	Is courteous and respectful at all times.		
22.	Reports any changes in resident to the nurse. Documents procedure using facility guidelines.		

_____   _____
Date Reviewed   Instructor Signature

_____   _____
Date Performed   Instructor Signature

Giving a cleansing enema

		yes	no
1.	Identifies self by name. Identifies resident. Greets resident by name.		
2.	Washes hands.		
3.	Explains procedure to resident. Speaks clearly, slowly, and directly. Maintains face-to-face contact whenever possible.		
4.	Provides for resident's privacy with a curtain, screen, or door.		
5.	Adjusts bed to a safe level, usually waist high. Locks bed wheels.		
6.	Helps resident into left-sided Sims' position. Covers with a bath blanket.		
7.	Places IV pole beside the bed. Raises the side rail.		

8.	Clamps enema tube. Prepares the enema solution. Adds specific additive, if ordered. Fills bag with 500-1000 mL of warm water and swishes fluid to mix well. Checks water temperature with bath thermometer.		
9.	Unclamps tube. Lets a small amount of solution run through the tubing to release the air. Re-clamps tube.		
10.	Hangs bag on IV pole. Using the tape measure, makes sure bottom of enema bag is not more than 12 inches above resident's anus.		
11.	Puts on gloves.		
12.	Places bed protector under resident. Asks resident to remove undergarments or helps him do so. Places bedpan close to resident's body.		
13.	Lubricates two to four inches of the tip of the tubing with lubricating jelly.		
14.	Asks resident to breathe deeply.		
15.	Places one hand on upper buttock. Lifts to expose the anus. Asks resident to take a deep breath and exhale. Using other hand, inserts tip of the tubing two to four inches into the rectum. Stops immediately if resistance is felt or if the resident complains of pain.		
16.	Unclamps tubing. Allows solution to flow slowly into the rectum. Asks resident to take slow, deep breaths. Encourages him or her to take as much of the solution as possible.		
17.	Clamps tubing before the bag is empty when the solution is almost gone. Removes tip from rectum. Places tip into the enema bag. Does not contaminate self, resident, or bed linens.		

18.	Asks resident to hold the solution inside as long as possible.		
19.	Helps resident to use bedpan, commode, or get to the bathroom. Raises head of the bed, if resident is using bedpan. If resident uses a commode or bathroom, puts on robe and non-skid footwear. Lowers bed to its lowest position before resident gets up.		
20.	Removes and discards gloves. Washes hands.		
21.	Places toilet paper and washcloths or wipes within resident's reach. Asks resident to clean his hands with a hand wipe when finished, if he is able. If the resident is using the bathroom, asks him not to flush the toilet when finished.		
22.	Places call light within resident's reach. Washes hands. Asks resident to signal when finished. Leaves room.		
23.	When called by the resident, returns and washes hands. Puts on clean gloves.		
24.	Lowers head of the bed, if raised. Makes sure resident is still covered. Does not overexpose the resident.		
25.	Removes bedpan carefully and gently. Covers bedpan. Removes bed protector.		
26.	Gives perineal care if help is needed. Wipes from front to back. Dries perineal area with a towel. Helps resident put on undergarment. Places towel in a hamper or bag, and discards disposable supplies.		
27.	Takes bedpan to the bathroom. Calls nurse to observe enema results, whether in bedpan or in toilet. Empties contents into toilet.		
28.	Flushes toilet. Places bedpan in proper area for cleaning or cleans and stores it according to policy.		
29.	Removes and discards gloves. Washes hands.		
30.	Makes resident comfortable.		
31.	Returns bed to lowest position. Removes privacy measures.		
32.	Leaves call light within resident's reach.		
33.	Washes hands.		
34.	Is courteous and respectful at all times.		
35.	Reports any changes in resident to the nurse. Documents procedure using facility guidelines.		

_____   _____
Date Reviewed   Instructor Signature

_____   _____
Date Performed   Instructor Signature

Giving a commercial enema

		yes	no
1.	Identifies self by name. Identifies resident. Greets resident by name.		
2.	Washes hands.		
3.	Explains procedure to resident. Speaks clearly, slowly, and directly. Maintains face-to-face contact whenever possible.		
4.	Provides for resident's privacy with a curtain, screen, or door.		
5.	Adjusts bed to a safe level, usually waist high. Locks bed wheels.		
6.	Helps resident into left-sided Sims' position. Covers with a bath blanket.		
7.	Puts on gloves.		

8.	Places bed protector under resident. Asks resident to remove undergarments or helps him do so. Places bedpan close to resident's body.		
9.	Uncovers resident enough to expose anus only.		
10.	Adds extra lubricating jelly to the tip of bottle if needed.		
11.	Asks resident to breathe deeply to relieve cramps during procedure.		
12.	Places one hand on the upper buttock. Lifts to expose anus. Asks resident to take a deep breath and exhale. Using other hand, inserts tip of the tubing about one and a half inches into the rectum. Stops immediately if resistance is felt or if the resident complains of pain.		
13.	Slowly squeezes and rolls the enema container so that solution runs inside resident. Stops when container is almost empty.		
14.	Removes tip from rectum, continuing to keep pressure on the container until bottle is placed inside the box upside down.		
15.	Asks resident to hold solution inside as long as possible.		
16.	Helps resident to use bedpan, commode, or go to the bathroom. Raises head of bed, if resident is using bedpan. If the resident uses a commode or bathroom, puts on robe and non-skid footwear. Lowers bed to its lowest position before resident gets up.		
17.	Removes and discards gloves. Washes hands.		

18.	Places toilet paper and washcloths or wipes within resident's reach. Asks resident to clean his hands with a hand wipe when finished, if he is able. If resident is using the bathroom, asks him not to flush toilet when finished.		
19.	Places call light within resident's reach. Washes hands. Asks resident to signal when finished. Leaves room.		
20.	When called by resident, returns and washes hands. Puts on clean gloves.		
21.	Lowers head of the bed, if raised. Makes sure resident is still covered. Does not overexpose the resident.		
22.	Removes bedpan carefully. Covers bedpan. Removes bed protector.		
23.	Gives perineal care if help is needed. Wipes from front to back. Dries perineal area with a towel. Helps resident put on undergarment. Places towel in a hamper or bag, and discards disposable supplies.		
24.	Takes bedpan to bathroom. Calls nurse to observe enema results, whether in bedpan or in toilet. Empties contents into toilet.		
25.	Flushes toilet. Places bedpan in proper area for cleaning or cleans and stores it according to policy.		
26.	Removes and discards gloves. Washes hands.		
27.	Makes resident comfortable.		
28.	Returns bed to lowest position. Removes privacy measures.		
29.	Leaves call light within resident's reach.		
30.	Washes hands.		
31.	Is courteous and respectful at all times.		

| 32. | Reports any changes in resident to the nurse. Documents procedure using facility guidelines. | | |

_____   _____
Date Reviewed   Instructor Signature

_____   _____
Date Performed   Instructor Signature

Collecting a stool specimen

		yes	no
1.	Identifies self by name. Identifies resident. Greets resident by name.		
2.	Washes hands.		
3.	Explains procedure to resident. Speaks clearly, slowly, and directly. Maintains face-to-face contact whenever possible.		
4.	Provides for resident's privacy with a curtain, screen, or door.		
5.	Puts on gloves.		
6.	When resident is ready to move bowels, asks him not to urinate at the same time. Asks him not to put toilet paper in with sample. Provides a plastic bag for toilet paper.		
7.	Fits hat to toilet or commode, or provides resident with bedpan. Places toilet paper and washcloths or wipes within resident's reach. Asks resident to clean his hands with a hand wipe when finished, if he is able.		
8.	Asks resident to signal when he is finished with bowel movement. Makes sure call light is within reach.		
9.	Removes and discards gloves. Washes hands. Leaves room.		
10.	When called by the resident, returns and washes hands. Puts on clean gloves.		
11.	Gives perineal care if help is needed.		

12.	Using two tongue blades, takes about two tablespoons of stool and puts it in container. Covers it tightly, applies label, and places specimen in a clean plastic bag.		
13.	Wraps tongue blades in toilet paper and places them in plastic bag with used toilet paper. Discards bag in proper container. Empties bedpan or container into toilet. Flushes toilet. Places in proper area for cleaning or cleans it according to facility policy.		
14.	Removes and discards gloves. Washes hands.		
15.	Makes resident comfortable.		
16.	Returns bed to lowest position. Removes privacy measures.		
17.	Leaves call light within resident's reach.		
18.	Washes hands.		
19.	Is courteous and respectful at all times.		
20.	Reports any changes in resident to the nurse. Documents procedure using facility guidelines. Takes specimen and lab slip to designated place promptly.		

_____   _____
Date Reviewed   Instructor Signature

_____   _____
Date Performed   Instructor Signature

Testing a stool specimen for occult blood

		yes	no
1.	Washes hands.		
2.	Puts on gloves.		
3.	Opens test card.		
4.	Picks up a tongue blade. Gets small amount of stool from specimen container.		

5.	Using a tongue blade, smears a small amount of stool onto Box A of test card.		
6.	Flips tongue blade (or uses new tongue blade). Gets some stool from another part of specimen. Smears small amount of stool onto Box B of test card.		
7.	Closes test card. Turns over to other side.		
8.	Opens flap.		
9.	Opens developer. Applies developer to each box. Follows manufacturer's instructions.		
10.	Waits amount of time listed in instructions, usually between 10 and 60 seconds.		
11.	Watches squares for any color changes. Records color changes. Follows instructions.		
12.	Places tongue blade(s) and test packet in plastic bag.		
13.	Disposes of plastic bag properly in biohazard container.		
14.	Removes and discards gloves.		
15.	Washes hands.		
16.	Documents procedure using facility guidelines. Reports results to the nurse.		

_____   _____
Date Reviewed   Instructor Signature

_____   _____
Date Performed   Instructor Signature

Caring for an ostomy

		yes	no
1.	Identifies self by name. Identifies resident. Greets resident by name.		
2.	Washes hands.		
3.	Explains procedure to resident. Speaks clearly, slowly, and directly. Maintains face-to-face contact whenever possible.		

4.	Provides for resident's privacy with a curtain, screen, or door.		
5.	Adjusts bed to safe working level, usually waist high. Locks bed wheels. Raises head of bed.		
6.	Puts on gloves.		
7.	Places bed protector under resident. Covers resident with a bath blanket. Pulls down top sheet and blankets. Exposes only ostomy site. Offers resident a towel to keep clothing dry.		
8.	Undoes ostomy belt if used. Pulls on one edge of ostomy appliance to release air.		
9.	Removes ostomy bag carefully. Places it in plastic bag. Notes color, odor, consistency, and amount of stool in the bag.		
10.	Wipes area around stoma with toilet paper or gauze. Discards paper/gauze in plastic bag.		
11.	Adds small amount of mild soap or cleanser to the warm water. Using a washcloth, washes area gently in one direction, away from the stoma. Rinses. Pats dry with another towel. Applies skin barrier as ordered. Temporarily covers stoma opening with gauze squares.		
12.	Applies deodorant to bag if used. Removes gauze squares, and places in plastic bag. Puts clean ostomy drainage bag on resident. Holds in place and seals securely. Makes sure bottom of the bag is clamped. Attaches to ostomy belt if used.		
13.	Removes bed protector and discards. Places soiled linens in proper container.		
14.	Removes bag and gauze squares. Discards bag and squares in proper container.		
15.	Removes and discards gloves. Washes hands.		

		yes	no
16.	Makes resident comfortable.		
17.	Returns bed to lowest position. Removes privacy measures.		
18.	Leaves call light within resident's reach.		
19.	Washes hands.		
20.	Is courteous and respectful at all times.		
21.	Reports any changes in resident to the nurse. Documents procedure using facility guidelines.		

_____   _____
Date Reviewed   Instructor Signature

_____   _____
Date Performed   Instructor Signature

16
The Urinary System

Providing catheter care			
		yes	no
1.	Identifies self by name. Identifies resident. Greets resident by name.		
2.	Washes hands.		
3.	Explains procedure to resident. Speaks clearly, slowly, and directly. Maintains face-to-face contact whenever possible.		
4.	Provides for resident's privacy with a curtain, screen, or door.		
5.	Adjusts bed to a safe level. Locks bed wheels.		
6.	Lowers head of bed. Positions resident lying flat on her back.		
7.	Removes or folds back top bedding. Keeps resident covered with bath blanket.		
8.	Tests water temperature with thermometer or wrist and ensures it is safe. Has resident check water temperature. Adjusts if necessary.		
9.	Puts on gloves.		

10.	Avoids contact with clothing and soiled pads or soiled linens throughout procedure.		
11.	Asks resident to flex her knees and raise buttocks off the bed by pushing against mattress with her feet. Places clean bed protector under her buttocks.		
12.	Exposes only area necessary to clean the catheter.		
13.	Places towel or pad under catheter tubing before washing.		
14.	Applies soap to wet washcloth. If a male resident is uncircumcised, pulls back foreskin first. Cleans area around meatus. Uses a clean area of washcloth for each stroke.		
15.	Holds catheter near meatus. Avoids tugging catheter.		
16.	Cleans at least four inches of catheter nearest meatus. Moves in only one direction, away from meatus. Uses a clean area of cloth for each stroke.		
17.	Rinses area around meatus, using a clean area of washcloth for each stroke. Pats dry with clean cloth.		
18.	Rinses at least four inches of catheter nearest meatus. Moves in only one direction, away from meatus. Uses a clean area of the cloth for each stroke.		
19.	Removes bed protector and discards. Removes towel or pad from under catheter tubing and places in proper containers.		
20.	Empties basin in toilet and flushes toilet. Places in proper area for cleaning or returns to storage.		
21.	Removes gloves and discards. Washes hands.		
22.	Replaces top covers. Removes bath blanket. Makes resident comfortable.		

23.	Returns bed to lowest position. Removes privacy measures.		
24.	Leaves call light within resident's reach.		
25.	Washes hands.		
26.	Is courteous and respectful at all times.		
27.	Reports any changes in resident to the nurse. Documents procedure using facility guidelines.		

Date Reviewed _____ Instructor Signature

Date Performed _____ Instructor Signature

Emptying a catheter drainage bag

		yes	no
1.	Identifies self by name. Identifies resident. Greets resident by name.		
2.	Washes hands.		
3.	Explains procedure to resident. Speaks clearly, slowly, and directly. Maintains face-to-face contact whenever possible.		
4.	Provides for resident's privacy with a curtain, screen, or door.		
5.	Puts on gloves.		
6.	Places graduate on paper towel on the floor.		
7.	Opens drain or clamp on bag. Allows urine to flow out of bag into graduate. Does not let spout or clamp touch graduate.		
8.	When urine has drained, closes clamp. Using alcohol wipe, cleans drain clamp. Replaces drain in its holder on bag.		
9.	Goes into bathroom. Places graduate on a flat surface and measures at eye level. Notes amount and appearance of urine. Empties urine into toilet and flushes toilet.		

10.	Places container in area for cleaning or cleans and stores it according to policy. Discards paper towel.		
11.	Removes and discards gloves. Washes hands.		
12.	Leaves call light within resident's reach.		
13.	Washes hands.		
14.	Is courteous and respectful at all times.		
15.	Reports any changes in resident to the nurse. Documents procedure and amount of urine (output) using facility guidelines.		

Date Reviewed _____ Instructor Signature

Date Performed _____ Instructor Signature

Changing a condom catheter

		yes	no
1.	Identifies self by name. Identifies resident. Greets resident by name.		
2.	Washes hands.		
3.	Explains procedure to resident. Speaks clearly, slowly, and directly. Maintains face-to-face contact whenever possible.		
4.	Provides for resident's privacy with a curtain, screen, or door.		
5.	Adjusts bed to a safe level, usually waist high. Locks bed wheels.		
6.	Lowers head of bed. Positions resident lying flat on his back.		
7.	Removes or folds back top bedding. Keeps resident covered with bath blanket.		
8.	Puts on gloves.		
9.	Places clean bed protector under his buttocks.		
10.	Adjusts bath blanket to expose only genital area.		

11.	Removes condom catheter. Disconnects condom from tube and immediately caps tube. Does not allow tube to touch anything. Places condom and tape in the plastic bag.		
12.	Helps as necessary with perineal care.		
13.	Moves pubic hair away from penis so it does not get rolled into the condom.		
14.	Holds penis firmly. Places condom at tip of penis. Rolls towards base of penis. Leaves at least one inch of space between the drainage tip and glans of penis to prevent irritation. If resident is not circumcised, makes sure that foreskin is in normal position.		
15.	Secures condom to penis with special tape provided or uses self-adhesive. Applies in a spiral.		
16.	Connects catheter tip to drainage tubing. Does not touch tip to any object but drainage tubing. Makes sure tubing is not twisted or kinked.		
17.	Checks to see if collection bag is secured to leg. Makes sure drain is closed.		
18.	Removes bed protector and discards. Disposes of plastic bag properly. Places soiled clothing and linens in proper containers.		
19.	Cleans and stores supplies.		
20.	Removes and discards gloves. Washes hands.		
21.	Replaces top covers. Removes bath blanket. Makes resident comfortable.		
22.	Returns bed to lowest position. Removes privacy measures.		
23.	Leaves call light within resident's reach.		
24.	Washes hands.		

25.	Is courteous and respectful at all times.		
26.	Reports any changes in resident to the nurse. Documents procedure using facility guidelines.		

_____   _____
Date Reviewed   Instructor Signature

_____   _____
Date Performed   Instructor Signature

Collecting a routine urine specimen

		yes	no
1.	Identifies self by name. Identifies resident. Greets resident by name.		
2.	Washes hands.		
3.	Explains procedure to resident. Speaks clearly, slowly, and directly. Maintains face-to-face contact whenever possible.		
4.	Provides for resident's privacy with a curtain, screen, or door.		
5.	Puts on gloves.		
6.	Helps resident to the bathroom or commode, or offers bedpan or urinal.		
7.	Has resident void into "hat," urinal, or bedpan. Asks resident not to put toilet paper or stool in with the sample. Provides a plastic bag to discard toilet paper.		
8.	Places toilet paper and washcloths or wipes within resident's reach. Asks resident to clean his hands with a hand wipe when finished, if he is able.		
9.	Asks resident to signal when he is finished. Makes sure call light is within reach.		
10.	Removes and discards gloves. Washes hands. Leaves room.		
11.	When called, returns and washes hands. Puts on clean gloves.		

		yes	no
12.	Gives perineal care if help is needed.		
13.	Takes bedpan, urinal, or commode pail to bathroom.		
14.	Pours urine into specimen container until container is at least half full.		
15.	Covers urine container with its lid. Does not touch inside of container. Wipes off outside with a paper towel and discards. Applies label, and places in clean plastic bag.		
16.	If using a bedpan or urinal, discards extra urine in the toilet. Flushes toilet. Places in proper area for cleaning or cleans it according to policy.		
17.	Removes and discards gloves. Washes hands.		
18.	Makes resident comfortable.		
19.	Returns bed to lowest position. Removes privacy measures.		
20.	Leaves call light within resident's reach.		
21.	Washes hands.		
22.	Is courteous and respectful at all times.		
23.	Reports any changes in resident to the nurse. Documents procedure using facility guidelines. Takes specimen and lab slip to designated place promptly.		

_____   _____
Date Reviewed   Instructor Signature

_____   _____
Date Performed   Instructor Signature

Collecting a clean-catch (mid-stream) urine specimen

		yes	no
1.	Identifies self by name. Identifies resident. Greets resident by name.		
2.	Washes hands.		
3.	Explains procedure to resident. Speaks clearly, slowly, and directly. Maintains face-to-face contact whenever possible.		
4.	Provides for resident's privacy with a curtain, screen, or door.		
5.	Puts on gloves.		
6.	Opens specimen kit. Does not touch inside of container or lid.		
7.	Cleans perineal area if resident cannot do it.		
8.	Asks resident to urinate a small amount into the bedpan, urinal, or toilet, and to stop before urination is complete.		
9.	Places container under urine stream. Does not touch resident's body with container. Has resident start urinating again. Fills container at least half full. Has resident stop urinating and removes container if possible. Has resident finish urinating in bedpan, urinal, or toilet.		
10.	After urination, gives perineal care if help is needed. Asks resident to clean his hands with hand wipes, if he is able.		
11.	Covers urine container with its lid. Does not touch inside of container. Wipes off outside with a paper towel and discards. Applies label, and places in clean plastic bag.		
12.	If using a bedpan or urinal, discards extra urine in the toilet. Flushes toilet. Places in proper area for cleaning or cleans it according to policy.		
13.	Removes and discards gloves. Washes hands.		
14.	Makes resident comfortable.		
15.	Returns bed to lowest position. Removes privacy measures.		

Name: _____

16.	Leaves call light within resident's reach.		
17.	Washes hands.		
18.	Is courteous and respectful at all times.		
19.	Reports any changes in resident to the nurse. Documents procedure using facility guidelines. Takes specimen and lab slip to designated place promptly.		

_____   _____
Date Reviewed   Instructor Signature

_____   _____
Date Performed   Instructor Signature

Collecting a 24-hour urine specimen

		yes	no
1.	Identifies self by name. Identifies resident. Greets resident by name.		
2.	Washes hands.		
3.	Explains procedure to resident. Speaks clearly, slowly, and directly. Maintains face-to-face contact whenever possible. Emphasizes that all urine must be saved. Asks resident not to put toilet paper or stool in with the sample.		
4.	Provides for resident's privacy with a curtain, screen, or door.		
5.	Places a sign near the resident's bed to let all care team members know that a 24-hour specimen is being collected.		
6.	When starting the collection, has resident completely empty the bladder. Discards urine. Notes exact time of this voiding. The collection will run until the same time the next day.		
7.	Washes hands and puts on gloves each time the resident voids. Measures I&O each time if needed.		

8.	Pours urine from bedpan, urinal, or hat into the container. Follows facility policy regarding storing container.		
9.	After each voiding, gives perineal care if help is needed. Asks resident to clean his hands with a hand wipe, if he is able.		
10.	Cleans equipment after each voiding.		
11.	Removes and discards gloves.		
12.	Washes hands.		
13.	After the last void of the 24-hour period, adds urine to specimen container. Removes sign.		
14.	Makes resident comfortable.		
15.	Returns bed to lowest position. Removes privacy measures.		
16.	Leaves call light within resident's reach.		
17.	Washes hands.		
18.	Is courteous and respectful at all times.		
19.	Reports any changes in resident to the nurse. Documents procedure using facility guidelines. Takes specimen containers and lab slip to designated place promptly.		

_____   _____
Date Reviewed   Instructor Signature

_____   _____
Date Performed   Instructor Signature

Testing urine with reagent strips

		yes	no
1.	Washes hands.		
2.	Puts on gloves.		
3.	Places paper towel on surface before setting urine specimen down.		
4.	Takes a strip from the bottle and recaps bottle. Closes it tightly.		
5.	Dips strip into specimen.		

6.	Follows manufacturer's instructions for when to remove strip. Removes strip at correct time.		
7.	Follows manufacturer's instructions for how long to wait after removing strip. After proper time has passed, compares strip with color chart on bottle. Does not touch bottle with strip.		
8.	Reads results.		
9.	Discards used items. Discards specimen in the toilet. Flushes toilet.		
10.	Removes and discards gloves.		
11.	Washes hands.		
12.	Records and reports results. Documents procedure using facility guidelines.		

_____   _____
Date Reviewed   Instructor Signature

_____   _____
Date Performed   Instructor Signature

17
The Reproductive System

Giving a vaginal irrigation			
		yes	no
1.	Identifies self by name. Identifies resident. Greets resident by name.		
2.	Washes hands.		
3.	Explains procedure to resident. Speaks clearly, slowly, and directly. Maintains face-to-face contact whenever possible.		
4.	Provides for resident's privacy with a curtain, screen, or door.		
5.	Adjusts bed to a safe level, usually waist high. Locks bed wheels.		
6.	Lowers head of bed. Positions resident lying flat on her back.		
7.	Puts on gloves.		

8.	Covers resident with a bath blanket. Asks her to hold it while pulling down top covers underneath. Does not expose more of her than is necessary.		
9.	Places a bed protector under resident's buttocks and hips.		
10.	Hangs prepared vaginal irrigation bag on IV pole and lowers pole so that bag is 12 inches above resident's perineal area.		
11.	Removes resident's underpants, exposing only as much of the resident's body as necessary.		
12.	Places bedpan under resident and makes sure she is in the dorsal recumbent position.		
13.	Opens clamp and allows a little water to run from tubing into bedpan to clear air from tubing.		
14.	Lubricates tip of tubing, if not already lubricated.		
15.	Inserts nozzle slowly and gently into vagina about two to three inches.		
16.	Begins slow flow of water or fluid by releasing clamp. Before vaginal irrigation bag is empty, clamps tubing.		
17.	Removes tubing slowly and gently and places tubing tip inside top of bag.		
18.	Raises head of the bed so that resident is in a semi-sitting position on the bedpan so that solution can drain.		
19.	After solution has drained into bedpan, removes bedpan and covers it. Removes bed protector and discards.		
20.	Brings bedpan to bathroom and checks contents for anything unusual. Empties bedpan unless nurse needs to check contents.		
21.	Flushes toilet. Places bedpan in area for cleaning or cleans and stores it according to policy.		

		yes	no
22.	Places soiled linens and clothing in proper containers.		
23.	Removes and discards gloves. Washes hands.		
24.	Puts clothing back on. Removes bath blanket and replaces top covers. Makes resident comfortable.		
25.	Returns bed to lowest position. Removes privacy measures.		
26.	Leaves call light within resident's reach.		
27.	Washes hands.		
28.	Is courteous and respectful at all times.		
29.	Reports any changes in resident to the nurse. Documents procedure using facility guidelines.		

_____   _____
Date Reviewed   Instructor Signature

_____   _____
Date Performed   Instructor Signature

18
The Integumentary System

Applying warm moist compresses			
		yes	no
1.	Identifies self by name. Identifies resident. Greets resident by name.		
2.	Washes hands.		
3.	Explains procedure to resident. Speaks clearly, slowly, and directly. Maintains face-to-face contact whenever possible.		
4.	Provides for resident's privacy with a curtain, screen, or door.		
5.	Fills basin one-half to two-thirds with warm water. Tests water temperature with thermometer or wrist. Ensures it is safe. Has resident check water temperature. Adjusts if necessary.		

		yes	no
6.	Soaks washcloth in the water. Wrings it out. Applies it to area needing a warm compress. Notes time. Quickly covers washcloth with plastic wrap and towel to keep it warm.		
7.	Checks area every five minutes. Removes compress if area is red or numb or if resident has pain or discomfort. Changes compress if cooling occurs. Removes compress after 20 minutes.		
8.	Removes privacy measures. Makes resident comfortable.		
9.	Empties, rinses, and wipes basin. Returns to proper storage. Discards plastic wrap.		
10.	Places soiled clothing and linens in appropriate containers.		
11.	Leaves call light within resident's reach.		
12.	Washes hands.		
13.	Is courteous and respectful at all times.		
14.	Reports any changes in resident to the nurse. Documents procedure using facility guidelines.		

_____   _____
Date Reviewed   Instructor Signature

_____   _____
Date Performed   Instructor Signature

Administering warm soaks			
		yes	no
1.	Identifies self by name. Identifies resident. Greets resident by name.		
2.	Washes hands.		
3.	Explains procedure to resident. Speaks clearly, slowly, and directly. Maintains face-to-face contact whenever possible.		

4.	Provides for resident's privacy with a curtain, screen, or door.		
5.	Fills basin half full of warm water. Tests water temperature with thermometer or wrist, and ensures it is safe. Has resident check water temperature. Adjusts if necessary.		
6.	Immerses body part in basin. Pads edge of the basin with a towel if needed. Uses a bath blanket to cover resident if needed for extra warmth.		
7.	Checks water temperature every five minutes. Adds warm water as needed to maintain temperature. Observes area for redness. Discontinues soak if resident has pain or discomfort.		
8.	Soaks for 15-20 minutes, or as ordered.		
9.	Removes basin. Uses towel to dry resident.		
10.	Removes privacy measures. Makes resident comfortable.		
11.	Empties, rinses, and wipes basin. Returns to proper storage.		
12.	Places soiled clothing and linens in appropriate containers.		
13.	Leaves call light within resident's reach.		
14.	Washes hands.		
15.	Is courteous and respectful at all times.		
16.	Reports any changes in resident to the nurse. Documents procedure using facility guidelines.		

_____   _____
Date Reviewed   Instructor Signature

_____   _____
Date Performed   Instructor Signature

Applying an Aquamatic K-Pad®		yes	no
1.	Identifies self by name. Identifies resident. Greets resident by name.		
2.	Washes hands.		
3.	Explains procedure to resident. Speaks clearly, slowly, and directly. Maintains face-to-face contact whenever possible.		
4.	Provides for resident's privacy with a curtain, screen, or door.		
5.	Makes sure surface on the bedside table is dry. Places control unit on bedside table. Makes sure cords are not frayed or damaged. Checks that tubing between pad and unit is intact.		
6.	Removes cover of control unit to check level of water. If it is low, fills it with distilled water to fill line.		
7.	Puts cover of control unit back in place.		
8.	Plugs unit in. Turns unit on.		
9.	Places pad in the cover. Does not pin pad to cover.		
10.	Uncovers area to be treated. Places covered pad. Notes time. Makes sure tubing is not hanging below bed. Makes sure tubing has no kinks.		
11.	Returns and checks area every five minutes. Removes pad if area is red or numb or if the resident reports pain or discomfort.		
12.	Checks water level. Refills with distilled water to fill line when necessary.		
13.	Turns off unit and removes pad after 20 minutes.		
14.	Removes privacy measures. Makes resident comfortable.		
15.	Cleans K-pad® according to instructions and returns to storage.		

16.	Places used linen in appropriate container.		
17.	Leaves call light within resident's reach.		
18.	Washes hands.		
19.	Is courteous and respectful at all times.		
20.	Reports any changes in resident to the nurse. Documents procedure using facility guidelines.		

_____   _____
Date Reviewed   Instructor Signature

_____   _____
Date Performed   Instructor Signature

Assisting with a sitz bath

		yes	no
1.	Identifies self by name. Identifies resident. Greets resident by name.		
2.	Washes hands.		
3.	Explains procedure to resident. Speaks clearly, slowly, and directly. Maintains face-to-face contact whenever possible.		
4.	Provides for resident's privacy with a curtain, screen, or door.		
5.	Puts on gloves.		
6.	Fills sitz bath container two-thirds full with warm water. Places sitz bath on toilet seat. Checks water temperature using bath thermometer.		
7.	Helps resident undress and get seated on the sitz bath.		
8.	Stays with resident, or leaves the room, as ordered. Makes sure resident knows how to use the emergency pull cord in the bathroom if it is needed.		
9.	Helps resident off of the sitz bath after 20 minutes. Provides towels. Helps with dressing if needed.		

10.	Empties, rinses, and wipes sitz bath container. Returns to proper storage.		
11.	Places soiled clothing and linens in appropriate containers.		
12.	Removes and discards gloves. Washes hands.		
13.	Makes resident comfortable. Removes privacy measures.		
14.	Leaves call light within resident's reach.		
15.	Washes hands.		
16.	Is courteous and respectful at all times.		
17.	Reports any changes in resident to the nurse. Documents procedure using facility guidelines.		

_____   _____
Date Reviewed   Instructor Signature

_____   _____
Date Performed   Instructor Signature

Applying ice packs

		yes	no
1.	Identifies self by name. Identifies resident. Greets resident by name.		
2.	Washes hands.		
3.	Explains procedure to resident. Speaks clearly, slowly, and directly. Maintains face-to-face contact whenever possible.		
4.	Provides for resident's privacy with a curtain, screen, or door.		
5.	Fills plastic bag or ice pack one-half to two-thirds full with crushed ice. Seals bag. Removes excess air. Covers bag or ice pack with towel or cover.		
6.	Applies pack or bag to the area as ordered. Notes time. Uses another towel to cover bag if it is too cold.		

7.	Checks area after five minutes for blisters or pale, white, or gray skin. Stops treatment if resident reports numbness or pain.		
8.	Removes ice pack or bag after 20 minutes or as ordered.		
9.	Removes privacy measures. Makes resident comfortable.		
10.	Empties and stores ice pack.		
11.	Places used linen in appropriate container.		
12.	Leaves call light within resident's reach.		
13.	Washes hands.		
14.	Is courteous and respectful at all times.		
15.	Reports any changes in resident to the nurse. Documents procedure using facility guidelines.		

_____   _____
Date Reviewed   Instructor Signature

_____   _____
Date Performed   Instructor Signature

Assisting the nurse with changing a non-sterile dressing

		yes	no
1.	Identifies self by name. Identifies resident. Greets resident by name.		
2.	Washes hands.		
3.	Explains procedure to resident. Speaks clearly, slowly, and directly. Maintains face-to-face contact whenever possible.		
4.	Provides for resident's privacy with a curtain, screen, or door.		
5.	Cuts pieces of tape long enough to secure the dressing, as needed. Opens gauze square packages without touching the insides or the gauze. Places opened package on a clean, flat surface, if asked.		

6.	Puts on gloves.		
7.	Only exposes the area where the dressing will be changed. Disposes of used dressing in proper container.		
8.	Removes and discards gloves in plastic bag.		
9.	Washes hands.		
10.	Puts on new gloves. Assists nurse with applying fresh gauze over the wound and taping it in place, as needed.		
11.	Removes and discards gloves. Washes hands.		
12.	Makes resident comfortable. Removes privacy measures.		
13.	Leaves call light within resident's reach.		
14.	Washes hands.		
15.	Is courteous and respectful at all times.		
16.	Reports any changes in resident to the nurse. Documents procedure using facility guidelines.		

_____   _____
Date Reviewed   Instructor Signature

_____   _____
Date Performed   Instructor Signature

Applying sterile gloves

		yes	no
1.	Washes hands.		
2.	Using a clean, flat, dry surface, removes outer wrapper from gloves. Places inner wrapper on the clean surface. The word "Left" should be on the left side, and the word "Right" should be on the right side.		
3.	Slowly opens the inner wrapper, only touching the small flaps of the wrapper.		

4.	Picks up the first glove by bottom end of the cuff. Slips fingers into the glove without touching the outside of the glove.		
5.	Slips gloved hand into the second glove in the area under the cuff.		
6.	Slowly slips fingers of ungloved hand into the second glove, and pulls it completely over hand and wrist.		
7.	With gloved second hand, finishes pulling first glove up and over the wrist. Adjusts fingers if any adjustment is necessary.		
8.	If either glove has a tear in it, stops and starts again with the second set of sterile gloves.		
9.	Keeps gloved hands in front of self and above the level of waist at all times during the procedure.		
10.	Assists nurse with sterile procedure.		

_____   _____
Date Reviewed   Instructor Signature

_____   _____
Date Performed   Instructor Signature

19
The Circulatory or Cardiovascular System

Putting knee-high elastic stockings on a resident			
		yes	no
1.	Identifies self by name. Identifies resident. Greets resident by name.		
2.	Washes hands.		
3.	Explains procedure to resident. Speaks clearly, slowly, and directly. Maintains face-to-face contact whenever possible.		
4.	Provides for resident's privacy with a curtain, screen, or door.		

5.	Adjusts bed to safe working level, usually waist high. Locks bed wheels.		
6.	With resident lying in supine position, removes his or her socks, shoes, or slippers, and exposes one leg. Exposes no more than one leg at a time.		
7.	Takes one stocking and turns it inside-out at least to the heel area.		
8.	Places foot of stocking over toes, foot, and heel. Makes sure heel is in the right place (heel should be in heel of stocking).		
9.	Pulls top of stocking over foot, heel, and leg.		
10.	Makes sure there are no twists or wrinkles in stocking after it is on the leg.		
11.	Repeats steps 7 through 10 for the other leg.		
12.	Makes resident comfortable.		
13.	Returns bed to lowest position. Removes privacy measures.		
14.	Leaves call light within resident's reach.		
15.	Washes hands.		
16.	Is courteous and respectful at all times.		
17.	Reports any changes in resident to the nurse. Documents procedure using facility guidelines.		

_____   _____
Date Reviewed   Instructor Signature

_____   _____
Date Performed   Instructor Signature

20
The Respiratory System

Collecting a sputum specimen			
		yes	no
1.	Identifies self by name. Identifies resident. Greets resident by name.		

		yes	no
2.	Washes hands.		
3.	Explains procedure to resident. Speaks clearly, slowly, and directly. Maintains face-to-face contact whenever possible.		
4.	Provides for resident's privacy with a curtain, screen, or door.		
5.	Puts on mask and gloves.		
6.	Asks resident to rinse her mouth with water. Assists as necessary. Has her spit rinse water in the emesis basin, if she does not use the sink.		
7.	Asks resident to cough deeply, so that sputum comes up from the lungs. Gives resident tissues to cover her mouth. Asks resident to spit sputum into container.		
8.	When about two tablespoons of sputum have been obtained, covers container tightly. Wipes any sputum off the outside of the container with tissues. Discards tissues. Applies label and puts container in plastic bag and seals the bag.		
9.	Removes and discards gloves and mask. Washes hands.		
10.	Leaves call light within resident's reach.		
11.	Washes hands.		
12.	Is courteous and respectful at all times.		
13.	Reports any changes in resident to the nurse. Documents procedure using facility guidelines. Takes specimen container and lab slip to the designated place promptly.		

_____   _____
Date Reviewed   Instructor Signature

_____   _____
Date Performed   Instructor Signature

Assisting with deep breathing and coughing exercises

		yes	no
1.	Identifies self by name. Identifies resident. Greets resident by name.		
2.	Washes hands.		
3.	Explains procedure to resident. Speaks clearly, slowly, and directly. Maintains face-to-face contact whenever possible.		
4.	Provides for resident's privacy with a curtain, screen, or door.		
5.	Puts on gloves.		
6.	Positions resident in Fowler's position with a pillow over abdomen, if needed.		
7.	Asks her to wrap her arms around the pillow and hold pillow tightly against her abdomen.		
8.	Tells resident to take a deep breath and hold the breath for a few seconds.		
9.	Asks the resident to exhale for as long as possible through lips that are pursed.		
10.	Tells resident to then repeat the deep breathing exercise a few more times.		
11.	Makes sure tissues are nearby. Asks resident to hold the pillow tightly, breathe in once deeply, and then cough as forcefully as possible. Collects any secretions with the tissues and disposes of tissues temporarily in the emesis basin.		
12.	Repeats sequence above the designated number of times.		
13.	Disposes of tissues in nearest no-touch receptacle.		
14.	Cleans and stores emesis basin.		
15.	Removes and discards gloves. Washes hands.		
16.	Makes resident comfortable. Removes privacy measures.		

17.	Leaves call light within resident's reach.		
18.	Washes hands.		
19.	Is courteous and respectful at all times.		
20.	Reports any changes in resident to the nurse. Documents procedure using facility guidelines.		

_____   _____
Date Reviewed   Instructor Signature

_____   _____
Date Performed   Instructor Signature

21
The Musculoskeletal System

Applying elastic bandages		yes	no
1.	Identifies self by name. Identifies resident. Greets resident by name.		
2.	Washes hands.		
3.	Explains procedure to resident. Speaks clearly, slowly, and directly. Maintains face-to-face contact whenever possible.		
4.	Provides for resident's privacy with a curtain, screen, or door.		
5.	Adjusts bed to safe working level, usually waist high. Locks bed wheels.		
6.	Avoids trauma or pain to resident throughout procedure.		
7.	Assists resident to get into supine (flat on the back) position.		
8.	Exposes only the part to be bandaged.		
9.	Holds rolled bandage with one hand and, with the other hand, puts the loose end on top of extremity.		
10.	Wraps extremity, beginning at the spot furthest from the heart.		

11.	Wraps bandage once around the beginning spot, and turns over the tip so that an anchor is made.		
12.	Wraps one more time around the spot where the anchor lies, and then begins slowly wrapping in overlapping spirals up the extremity.		
13.	Smoothes out entire bandage, removing any wrinkles.		
14.	Secures bandage with self-closure, clip, safety pin, or tape.		
15.	Straightens all of the linens.		
16.	Removes and re-applies bandage as directed. Washes and dries bandages as necessary.		
17.	Makes resident comfortable.		
18.	Returns bed to lowest position. Removes privacy measures.		
19.	Leaves call light within resident's reach.		
20.	Washes hands.		
21.	Is courteous and respectful at all times.		
22.	Reports any changes in resident to the nurse. Documents procedure using facility guidelines.		

_____   _____
Date Reviewed   Instructor Signature

_____   _____
Date Performed   Instructor Signature

22
The Nervous System

Caring for eyeglasses		yes	no
1.	Identifies self by name. Identifies resident. Greets resident by name.		
2.	Washes hands.		
3.	Explains procedure to resident. Speaks clearly, slowly, and directly. Maintains face-to-face contact whenever possible.		

4.	Provides for resident's privacy with a curtain, screen, or door.		
5.	Removes eyeglasses and places in emesis basin.		
6.	Lines sink with towel.		
7.	Cleans eyeglasses over lined sink. Washes glass lenses in lukewarm water and rinses. Cleans plastic lenses with cleaning fluid and a lens cloth.		
8.	Dries with soft, 100% cotton cloth or special lens cloth. Does not dry with tissues, as they may scratch eyeglasses.		
9.	Assists resident to replace eyeglasses on face. Places over the ears and positions comfortably.		
10.	Makes resident comfortable. Removes privacy measures.		
11.	Leaves call light within resident's reach.		
12.	Washes hands.		
13.	Is courteous and respectful at all times.		
14.	Reports any changes in resident to the nurse. Documents procedure using facility guidelines.		

_____   _____
Date Reviewed   Instructor Signature

_____   _____
Date Performed   Instructor Signature

23
The Endocrine System

Providing foot care			
		yes	no
1.	Identifies self by name. Identifies resident. Greets resident by name.		
2.	Washes hands.		
3.	Explains procedure to resident. Speaks clearly, slowly, and directly. Maintains face-to-face contact whenever possible.		

4.	Provides for resident's privacy with a curtain, screen, or door.		
5.	If the resident is in bed, adjusts bed to lowest position. Locks bed wheels.		
6.	Fills basin halfway with warm water. Tests water temperature with thermometer or wrist. Ensures it is safe. Has resident check water temperature. Adjusts if necessary.		
7.	Places basin on the bath mat. Supports foot and ankle throughout procedure.		
8.	Removes resident's socks. Completely submerges resident's feet in water. Soaks feet for five to ten minutes.		
9.	Puts on gloves.		
10.	Removes one foot from water. Washes entire foot, including between the toes and around nail beds, with a soapy washcloth.		
11.	Rinses entire foot, including between the toes.		
12.	Using a towel, pats dry entire foot, including between the toes.		
13.	Repeats steps 10 through 12 for the other foot.		
14.	Puts lotion in hand. Warms lotion by rubbing hands together.		
15.	Massages lotion into feet (top and bottom), except between the toes, removing excess (if any) with a towel. Makes sure lotion has been absorbed and feet are completely dry.		
16.	Empties, rinses, and wipes basin. Returns to proper storage.		
17.	Disposes of soiled linen in the proper container.		
18.	Removes and discards gloves. Washes hands.		

		yes	no
19.	Assists resident to put on clean socks. Makes resident comfortable.		
20.	Removes privacy measures.		
21.	Leaves call light within resident's reach.		
22.	Washes hands.		
23.	Is courteous and respectful at all times.		
24.	Reports any changes in resident to the nurse. Documents procedure using facility guidelines.		

_____ _____
Date Reviewed   Instructor Signature

_____ _____
Date Performed   Instructor Signature

25
Rehabilitation and Restorative Care

Assisting with ambulation for a resident using a cane, walker, or crutches			
		yes	no
1.	Identifies self by name. Identifies resident. Greets resident by name.		
2.	Washes hands.		
3.	Explains procedure to resident. Speaks clearly, slowly, and directly. Maintains face-to-face contact whenever possible.		
4.	Provides for resident's privacy with a curtain, screen, or door.		
5.	Adjusts bed to a low position so that the resident's feet are flat on the floor. Locks bed wheels.		
6.	Puts non-skid footwear on resident and securely fastens.		
7.	Stands in front of and faces resident.		
8.	Places gait belt below the rib cage and above the waist. Does not put it over bare skin. Grasps belt securely on both sides.		

		yes	no
9.	Braces resident's lower legs with caregiver's legs to prevent slipping.		
10.	On the count of three, slowly helps resident to stand.		
11.	Helps as needed with ambulation with cane, walker, or crutches.		
12.	Walks slightly behind and on the weaker side of resident. Holds the gait belt, if one is used.		
13.	Watches for obstacles in the resident's path. Asks resident to look ahead, not down at his feet.		
14.	Encourages resident to rest if he is tired. Lets resident set the pace. Discusses how far he plans to go based on care plan.		
15.	After ambulation, removes gait belt. Makes resident comfortable.		
16.	If leaving the resident in bed, returns bed to lowest position. Removes privacy measures.		
17.	Leaves call light within resident's reach.		
18.	Washes hands.		
19.	Is courteous and respectful at all times.		
20.	Reports any changes in resident to the nurse. Documents procedure using facility guidelines.		

_____ _____
Date Reviewed   Instructor Signature

_____ _____
Date Performed   Instructor Signature

Assisting with passive range of motion exercises			
		yes	no
1.	Identifies self by name. Identifies resident. Greets resident by name.		
2.	Washes hands.		

3.	Explains procedure to resident. Speaks clearly, slowly, and directly. Maintains face-to-face contact whenever possible.		
4.	Provides for resident's privacy with a curtain, screen, or door.		
5.	Adjusts bed to a safe level, usually waist high. Locks bed wheels.		
6.	Positions resident lying supine on the bed. Positions body in good alignment.		
7.	Repeats each exercise at least three times.		
8.	**Shoulder**		
	Performs the following movements properly, supporting the resident's arm at the elbow and wrist by placing one hand under the elbow and the other hand under the wrist:		
	1. Extension		
	2. Flexion		
	3. Abduction		
	4. Adduction		
9.	**Elbow**		
	Performs the following movements properly, holding the wrist with one hand, and holding the elbow with the other:		
	1. Flexion		
	2. Extension		
	3. Pronation		
	4. Supination		
10.	**Wrist**		
	Performs the following movements properly, holding the wrist with one hand, and using the fingers of the other hand to help the joint through the motions:		
	1. Flexion		
	2. Dorsiflexion		
	3. Radial flexion		

	4. Ulnar flexion		
11.	**Thumb**		
	Performs the following movements properly:		
	1. Abduction		
	2. Adduction		
	3. Opposition		
	4. Flexion		
	5. Extension		
12.	**Fingers**		
	Performs the following movements properly:		
	1. Flexion		
	2. Extension		
	3. Abduction		
	4. Adduction		
13.	**Hip**		
	Performs the following movements properly, placing one hand under the knee and one under the ankle:		
	1. Abduction		
	2. Adduction		
	3. Internal rotation		
	4. External rotation		
14.	**Knees**		
	Performs the following movements properly, placing one hand under the knee and one under the ankle:		
	1. Flexion		
	2. Extension		
15.	**Ankles**		
	Performs the following movements properly, supporting the foot and ankle:		
	1. Dorsiflexion		
	2. Plantar flexion		
	3. Supination		
	4. Pronation		

16.	*Toes*		
	Performs the following movements properly:		
	1. Flexion		
	2. Extension		
	3. Abduction		
17.	While supporting the limbs, moves all joints gently, slowly, and smoothly through the range of motion to the point of resistance. Stops exercises if any pain occurs.		
18.	Returns bed to lowest position. Removes privacy measures.		
19.	Leaves call light within resident's reach.		
20.	Washes hands.		
21.	Is courteous and respectful at all times.		
22.	Reports any changes in resident to the nurse. Documents procedure using facility guidelines.		

_____   _____
Date Reviewed   Instructor Signature

_____   _____
Date Performed   Instructor Signature

5.	Removes nail polish from digits to be used for pulse oximetry, if necessary.		
6.	Removes sensor probe from package and places clip-on probe on finger, toe, or earlobe.		
7.	Turns on the device. The pulse oximetry reading should appear on the screen quickly.		
8.	Asks resident to not remove or adjust pulse oximetry device. Asks resident to press call signal if the device comes off or dislodges.		
9.	Makes resident comfortable.		
10.	Removes privacy measures.		
11.	Leaves call light within resident's reach.		
12.	Washes hands.		
13.	Is courteous and respectful at all times.		
14.	Reports any changes in resident to the nurse. Documents procedure using facility guidelines.		

_____   _____
Date Reviewed   Instructor Signature

_____   _____
Date Performed   Instructor Signature

26
Subacute Care

Applying a pulse oximetry device			
		yes	no
1.	Identifies self by name. Identifies resident. Greets resident by name.		
2.	Washes hands.		
3.	Explains procedure to resident. Speaks clearly, slowly, and directly. Maintains face-to-face contact whenever possible.		
4.	Provides for resident's privacy with a curtain, screen, or door.		

27
End-of-Life Care

Postmortem care			
		yes	no
1.	Identifies self by name. Identifies resident. Greets resident by name.		
2.	Washes hands.		
3.	Explains procedure to resident's family and asks them to step outside. Is courteous, respectful, and compassionate at all times.		

4.	Provides for privacy with a curtain, screen, or door.		
5.	Adjusts bed to safe working level, usually waist high. Locks bed wheels.		
6.	Avoids trauma to the resident's body throughout the procedure. Treats body with utmost respect.		
7.	Puts on gloves.		
8.	Turns off any oxygen, suction, or other equipment, if directed by the nurse. Does not remove any tubes or other equipment.		
9.	Closes eyes without pressure.		
10.	Positions body in good alignment, on the back with legs straight. Folds arms across the abdomen.		
11.	Closes mouth. Places rolled towel under the chin.		
12.	Gently bathes body. Is careful to avoid bruising. Replaces any dressings only if directed to do so.		
13.	Combs or brushes hair gently without tugging.		
14.	Places drainage pads where needed, usually under the head and/or under the perineal area and buttocks.		
15.	Puts a clean gown on the body.		
16.	Covers body to just over the shoulders with sheet. Does not cover face or head.		
17.	Tidies room so family may visit.		
18.	Removes all used supplies and linen.		
19.	Follows facility policy for handling or removing personal items.		
20.	Removes and discards gloves.		
21.	Washes hands.		

22.	Returns bed to low position if raised. Turns lights down and allows family to enter and spend private time with resident.		
23.	Returns after family departs and puts on clean gloves.		
24.	Places shroud on resident and follows instructions on completing ID tags.		
25.	Removes and discards gloves.		
26.	Washes hands.		
27.	Reports and records observations. Documents procedure using facility guidelines.		

_____   _____
Date Reviewed   Instructor Signature

_____   _____
Date Performed   Instructor Signature

Practice Exam

After a nursing assistant has completed an approved training program in his or her state, he or she is given a competency evaluation (a certification exam or test) in order to be certified to work in that state. This exam usually consists of both a written evaluation and a skills evaluation. Review the guidelines for taking exams located in the appendix of the textbook on page 498.

1. One task commonly assigned to nursing assistants is
   (A) Inserting and removing tubes
   (B) Changing sterile dressings
   (C) Helping residents with toileting needs
   (D) Prescribing medications to residents

2. When a resident refuses to let the nursing assistant take her blood pressure, the nursing assistant should
   (A) Tell the resident that she must have it taken to prevent a serious illness
   (B) Take the resident's blood pressure anyway
   (C) Tell the resident that if she does this, she will get a treat later
   (D) Report this to the nurse

3. If a nursing assistant suspects that a resident is being abused, he should
   (A) Report it to the nurse immediately
   (B) Confront the abuser
   (C) Keep watching until he is sure abuse is occurring
   (D) Ask the resident if he thinks he is being abused

4. One safety device that helps transfer residents is called a
   (A) Waist restraint
   (B) Posey vest
   (C) Transfer belt
   (D) Geriatric chair

5. A nursing assistant may share a resident's medical information with which of the following?
   (A) The resident's friends
   (B) Other members of the healthcare team
   (C) The nursing assistant's friends
   (D) The resident's roommate

6. Which of the following is an objective statement?
   (A) Mr. Harris has a rash on his back.
   (B) Mrs. Carpenter has been having headaches lately.
   (C) Mr. Jansson says his medication makes him nauseous.
   (D) Ms. Peters' knees hurt when she is walking.

7. When may a nursing assistant hit a resident?
   (A) When the resident becomes combative
   (B) When the resident threatens to hit the nursing assistant or someone else
   (C) Only if the resident hits the nursing assistant first
   (D) Never

8. When giving perineal care to a female resident, a nursing assistant should
   (A) Wipe from front to back
   (B) Wipe from back to front
   (C) Use the same section of the washcloth for cleaning each part
   (D) Wash the anal area before the perineal area

9. How many milliliters (mL) equal one ounce?
   (A) 40
   (B) 30
   (C) 60
   (D) 20

10. According to OBRA, nursing assistants must complete at least ___ hours of training and must pass a competency evaluation before they can be employed.
(A) 100
(B) 250
(C) 50
(D) 75

11. Call lights should be placed
(A) High on the wall over the head of the bed
(B) Inside the bedside stand
(C) On the floor
(D) Within the resident's reach

12. An ombudsman is a person who
(A) Is in charge of the human resources department
(B) Teaches nursing assistants how to perform ROM exercises
(C) Is a legal advocate for residents and helps protect their rights
(D) Creates special diets for residents

13. To best communicate with a resident who has a hearing impairment, the nursing assistant should
(A) Use short sentences and simple words
(B) Shout
(C) Approach the resident from behind
(D) Raise the pitch of her voice

14. Which temperature site is considered the most accurate?
(A) Rectal
(B) Oral
(C) Axillary
(D) Tympanic

15. Psychosocial needs include
(A) Need for activity
(B) Need for sleep and rest
(C) Need for love and acceptance
(D) Need for clothing and shelter

16. How should a standard bedpan be positioned?
(A) According to the resident's preference
(B) Wider end aligned with resident's buttocks
(C) Smaller end aligned with resident's buttocks
(D) Smaller end facing the resident's head

17. If a nursing assistant encounters a sexual situation between two consenting residents, he should
(A) Provide privacy
(B) Ask the residents to stop
(C) Tell a clergyperson
(D) Tell other residents

18. The single most important thing a nursing assistant can do to prevent the spread of disease is to
(A) Keep her fingernails short and clean
(B) Wash her hands
(C) Apply and use PPE correctly
(D) Practice Transmission-Based Precautions on every resident

19. With regard to a resident's toenails, a nursing assistant should
(A) Never cut them
(B) Cut them when the resident requests it
(C) Cut them daily
(D) File them into rounded edges

20. Most of the accidents in a facility are related to
(A) Burns and scalds
(B) Failing to identify residents before performing care or serving food
(C) Choking
(D) Falls

21. Symptoms of myocardial infarction that are experienced more often by women include
(A) Back, shoulder or jaw pain
(B) Dizziness and confusion
(C) Cold and clammy skin
(D) Anxiety and a sense of doom

22. One way a nursing assistant can help a new resident adjust to life in a facility is to
(A) Tell the resident how much work it is to care for him
(B) Hide any mistakes the nursing assistant makes so that the resident will feel more confident in her work
(C) Listen if the resident wants to express his feelings
(D) Push the resident to join in activities even if he does not want to because it is the best thing for him

23. In what order should range of motion exercises be performed?
    (A) Start from the feet and work up
    (B) Start from the head and work down
    (C) The arms and legs should be exercised first
    (D) The arms and legs should be exercised last

24. A bed made while the resident is in the bed is called a(n)
    (A) Open bed
    (B) Closed bed
    (C) Occupied bed
    (D) Surgical bed

25. When providing personal care, the nursing assistant should
    (A) Do the task for the resident if it seems like it will take him a long time to complete it
    (B) Provide privacy for the resident
    (C) Tell the resident about other residents' conditions to be social
    (D) Discuss personal problems to get the resident's advice

26. Observing for changes in residents' skin is especially important to help prevent
    (A) Falls
    (B) Pressure ulcers
    (C) Edema
    (D) Weight gain

27. Generally, the last sense to leave a dying person is the sense of
    (A) Sight
    (B) Taste
    (C) Smell
    (D) Hearing

28. If a nursing assistant cannot obtain a reading when measuring vital signs, she should
    (A) Record her best guess
    (B) Use the previous reading for that resident
    (C) Leave that space in the chart blank
    (D) Tell the nurse

29. At which site is body temperature most often taken?
    (A) Armpit (axillary)
    (B) Ear (tympanic)
    (C) Mouth (oral)
    (D) Rectum (rectal)

30. According to the USDA's MyPlate, which food groups should make up the largest proportion of the diet?
    (A) Vegetables and fruits
    (B) Proteins and grains
    (C) Grains and fruits
    (D) Dairy products and proteins

31. Normal changes of aging in the gastrointestinal system include
    (A) Increased ability to taste
    (B) More frequent constipation
    (C) Increased production of saliva and digestive fluids
    (D) Presence of blood or mucus in stool

32. To prevent dehydration, a nursing assistant should
    (A) Discourage fluids before bedtime
    (B) Withhold fluids so the resident will be really thirsty
    (C) Offer fresh water and other fluids often
    (D) Wake the resident during the night to offer fluids

33. A resident tells a nursing assistant that she is scared of dying. Which of the following would be the best response from the nursing assistant?
    (A) Reply, "If you attend church services more often, you probably won't be so afraid."
    (B) Listen quietly and ask questions when appropriate.
    (C) Tell the resident, "Don't worry so much. You won't be going anywhere soon."
    (D) Reply, "You might need to start taking new medication."

34. With catheters it is important for a nursing assistant to remember that
    (A) Tubing should be kinked
    (B) Perineal care does not need to be performed
    (C) The drainage bag should be kept lower than the hips or the bladder
    (D) The resident should lie on top of the tubing

35. If a nursing assistant sees a resident masturbating, the nursing assistant should
    (A) Run to the charge nurse and ask her what to do
    (B) Provide privacy for the resident
    (C) Tell the resident that he should not be doing that
    (D) Tell the other nursing assistants what happened

36. One way for a nursing assistant to promote normal urination is to
    (A) Reduce residents' intake of fluids
    (B) Discourage activity and exercise
    (C) Provide plenty of privacy and time for elimination
    (D) Ask residents to wait as long as they can before urinating so as to train the bladder to hold more fluids

37. When assisting a resident who has had a stroke, a nursing assistant should
    (A) Do everything for the resident
    (B) Lead with the stronger side when transferring
    (C) Dress the stronger side first
    (D) Place food in the affected, or weaker, side of the mouth

38. What does a diagnosis of prehypertension mean?
    (A) It means that the person has high blood pressure.
    (B) It means that the person does not have high blood pressure now but is likely to in the future.
    (C) It means that the person has low blood pressure.
    (D) It means that the person does not have low blood pressure now but is likely to in the future.

39. When should anti-embolic stockings be applied?
    (A) In the morning
    (B) In the afternoon
    (C) Right before the resident goes to bed
    (D) During or after surgery

40. Residents with COPD might be fearful of
    (A) Not being able to breathe
    (B) Not being able to walk
    (C) Not being able to eat
    (D) Not being able to remember friends and family members

41. A resident with tuberculosis must
    (A) Take as little of his prescribed medication as possible—just enough until symptoms disappear
    (B) Take all of the prescribed medication
    (C) Keep the doors to the airborne infection isolation room open
    (D) Use an inhaler

42. To best respond to a resident with Alzheimer's disease who is repeating a question over and over again, the nursing assistant should
    (A) Answer the question each time it is asked, using the same words
    (B) Try to silence the resident
    (C) Tell the resident to stop
    (D) Explain to the resident that he just asked that question

43. If a resident with Alzheimer's disease has hallucinations, a nursing assistant should
    (A) Ignore the hallucination and reassure the resident
    (B) Pretend to see what the resident is seeing
    (C) Tell the resident that she is imagining things
    (D) Tell the resident's family to see if they can get her to stop

44. Diabetes is more common in people who
    (A) Have a family history of the illness
    (B) Are under the age of 50
    (C) Are unable to get out of bed
    (D) Are underweight

45. HIV/AIDS can be transmitted by
    (A) Unprotected or poorly protected sexual contact with an infected person
    (B) Hugging an infected person
    (C) Drinking water from the same fountain as an infected person
    (D) Being bitten by a mosquito

46. A _____ tumor is non-cancerous; a _____ tumor is cancerous.
    (A) Malignant, benign
    (B) Benign, malignant
    (C) Malignant, metastasized
    (D) Metastasized, malignant

47. A nursing assistant must wear gloves when
    (A) Combing a resident's hair
    (B) Feeding a resident
    (C) Performing oral care
    (D) Performing range of motion exercises

48. To best communicate with a resident who has a vision impairment, the nursing assistant should
    (A) Rearrange furniture without telling the resident
    (B) Identify herself when she enters the room
    (C) Keep the lighting low at all times
    (D) Touch the resident before identifying herself

49. The first sign of skin breakdown is
    (A) Coolness
    (B) Bleeding
    (C) Discoloration
    (D) Numbness

50. What is the proper way to handle soiled bed linens?
    (A) Carry them away from the nursing assistant's body
    (B) Shake them in the air to get rid of contaminants
    (C) Take them into another resident's room
    (D) Put them on the nurses' desk until housekeeping picks them up